LIGHTEN UP!

with Louise Hagler

TASTY, LOW-FAT, LOW-CALORIE VEGETARIAN CUISINE

BOOK PUBLISHING COM

SUMMERTOWN, TENNE~

Cover and interior design by Louise Hagler
Cover photo by John Guider
Back Cover photo of Louise by Ina May Gaskin
Food Styling by Mary Ann Fowlkes and Louise Hagler

Book Publishing Company
PO Box 99
Summertown, TN 38483

ISBN 1-57067-011-0

Featured on the Cover, clockwise from top front to top back: POLENTA WITH ROASTED RED BELL PEPPER SAUCE, pg. 80, FAJITAS WITH TEXTURED VEGETABLE PROTEIN, pg. 109, THAI SLAW, pg. 37, LEMON TOFU CHEESECAKE, pg. 144, with FRESH MANGO SAUCE, pg. 151, and YELLOW, GREEN, AND ORANGE SVELTES, pg. 128.

Library of Congress Cataloging-in-Publication Data

Hagler, Louise
        Lighten Up! / With Louise Hagler.
                p.   cm.
        Includes index.
        ISBN 1-57067-011-0 (alk. paper)
        1. Vegetarian cookery.   I. Title.
RM236.H34   1995
641.5'636--dc20   95-21983
                                                   CIP

About the Nutritional Analyses in this book:

Calculations for the nutritional analyses in this book are based on the average number of servings listed with the recipes and the average amount of an ingredient, if a range is called for. Calculations are rounded up to the nearest gram. If two options for an ingredient are listed, the first one is used. Not included are optional ingredients, serving suggestions, or oil used for oiling pans, unless the amount is specified in the recipe.

TABLE OF CONTENTS

INTRODUCTION

This book presents the best of my search for a "light" but tantalizing vegetarian cuisine. Low-fat, low-calorie food can have all the taste and satisfaction you are looking for. Healthy food does not have to be "no fun" food. You don't have to give up flavor. These recipes range from familiar, comforting foods in a new reduced-fat and lower-calorie form, to innovative creations, which will entice your palate to new epicurean heights.

I love to cook and I love to eat. I have been a practicing and experimenting vegetarian for more than a quarter of a century. During this period of time I have changed the way I eat several times, according to need or new information. In the last few years I have been making a concerted effort to reduce the fat and calories in the food I prepare, while maintaining delicious flavor.

Most of the cooking I do is fairly quick and simple. All the recipes in this book are vegan; they contain no meat, eggs, or dairy products. Most of the ingredients are easy to find and may even be in your kitchen right now. Some of the foods may be new to you, such as tofu, tempeh, quinoa, jícama, arugula, vital wheat gluten, miso, textured vegetable protein, or kanten, but they should all be easy to find in your local natural food store or supermarket. Each section of this book will include some of these new and interesting foods that help make a well rounded vegan cuisine.

Good nutrition and good health go hand in hand. Numerous studies point toward a low-fat, low-calorie diet composed predominantly of whole grains, beans, vegetables and fruits as the key to maintaining good health. Moving away from the typical North American meat and dairy-based high-fat diet is a challenge. It requires retraining your taste buds, but you don't have to struggle with feelings of deprivation and frustration. Food preferences are acquired habits that can be changed with some planning and patience. The recipes in this book can help make it easy to switch to eating delicious low-fat, low-calorie foods.

As you trim the fat from your diet, remember that it takes time for the body to adjust to any changes. It takes about 6 weeks of consuming a low-fat, low-calorie diet for your body to stop craving the fatty foods you used to eat. Given the chance, the body will develop a preference for healthier foods. Help yourself by having easy to prepare, tasty, low-fat, low-calorie foods *readily available.*

As much as possible, I cook without oil. I use small amounts of oil in some of these recipes, usually olive or canola oil, for a hint of flavor and texture or to bring out the flavors of some herbs or spices that are only soluble in oil. In some cases, you can eliminate the oil and steam "sauté" in water, or add a couple of tablespoons of water to a small amount of oil. Using non-stick cookware helps make low-fat cooking possible.

Health experts are giving us many reasons to change to a low-fat, low-calorie diet that is high in fiber. *Only foods from the plant kingdom contain dietary fiber.* Whole grains and beans are the best sources. The fiber found in whole grains, beans, vegetables, and fruits helps to lower cholesterol levels as well as giving a feeling of "fullness." If cholesterol is a concern for you, remember, *there is no cholesterol in the plant kingdom.* Look for organic foods. It makes health-sense to eliminate pesticides and poisons from your life wherever possible.

If you are primarily interested in weight loss, keep in mind that slow and steady is the key to taking it off and keeping it off. If you consume a low-fat, low-calorie diet of primarily whole grains, beans, vegetables, and fruit, counting calories becomes unnecessary. Remember that when you eat, it takes about 20 minutes for your body to acknowledge that it has been fed. Train yourself to eat slowly, pausing frequently, chewing well, and enjoying every bite.

Exercise is an essential ingredient for both good health and weight loss, but always check with you doctor before beginning any new exercise program. You have to burn about 220 calories to take off 1 ounce of body fat or about 3500 calories to take off a pound. At 3 m.p.h., it takes 20 minutes of walking to burn 100 calories.

A general guideline to follow for maintaining a healthy diet is to keep your consumption of oil to between 10% and 20% of your total calories and consume around 40 grams of fiber a day. I try to keep a running count of the fat grams and calories I consume over a period of time and calculate the percentage of calories from fat in the total rather than with each individual food or meal. Sometimes my schedule does not allow me to eat the low-fat food I would prefer. So when I overdo on the fat grams at one meal, I make it up at the next meal or two by making the right choices. The nutritional analysis with each recipe in this book shows the amount of calories, protein, fat, carbohydrates, dietary fiber, and sodium in each serving.

So, go ahead, **LIGHTEN UP!**
Roll up sizzling **FAJITAS WITH TEXTURED VEGETABLE PROTEIN.**
Dip into creamy **TOFU-CILANTRO-GARLIC DIP.**
Delight in luscious **MINTED LENTIL SOUP.**
Savor some succulent **GLUTEN ROAST.**
Arouse your taste buds with **RIGATONI POBLANO.**
Enjoy the subtlety of **GREEN BEANS WITH SHIITAKE.**
Indulge in creamy **LEMON TOFU CHEESECAKE** with scrumptious **FRESH MANGO SAUCE** . . . *Happy and Healthy Cooking and Eating!*

SNACKS AND APPETIZERS

Be sure to keep a variety of these low-fat snacks and appetizers on hand. Try using crisp, raw, or lightly steamed VEGETABLES FOR DIPPING (pg. 27) to go with the creamy dips, spreads, and salsas that follow. It's an easy, delicious way to include more vegetables in your diet. Try some of the new fat-free and low-fat crackers or chips as dippers. Check the MAINLY BEANS section for more bean based "refries," pâtés, and spreads.

DIPS AND SPREADS

BABA GANOUJ

YIELD: 2½ CUPS

BABA GANOUJ is not limited to only eggplant for a base; any vegetable can be used. Butternut squash makes an excellent BABA GANOUJ.

2 lbs. eggplant, zucchini, or winter squash
2 Tbsp. fresh lemon juice
1 Tbsp. strong flavored olive oil
2 cloves garlic, minced
½ tsp. salt

1. Preheat the oven to 350°F.

2. Bake the eggplant or squash until soft (about 45 minutes to 1 hour). This can be done the day before.

3. When cool, cut in half, and scrape out of the skins. Blend in a food processor along with the rest of the ingredients. Serve with fat-free pita bread.

Per 2 Tbsp.: Calories: 19, Protein: 0 gm., Fat: 0 gm., Carbohydrates: 3 gm., Fiber: 1 gm., Sodium: 55 mg.

Fresh Shiitake Pâté or Spread

Yield: about 2 cups

This pâté or spread can be made with almost any kind of mushroom. We eat our fill of this and freeze the rest when our shiitake logs are fruiting abundantly.

1 Tbsp. olive oil
1 cup onion, chopped
1 clove garlic, pressed
½ lb. fresh shiitake, chopped (about 4 cups)
1 Tbsp. soy sauce
1 tsp. savory
½ tsp. thyme
¼ tsp. nutmeg
⅛ tsp. black pepper

1. Sauté the onion and garlic in the olive oil. When the onion starts to soften, add the shiitake, and cook over low heat about 5 minutes. Add the rest of the ingredients, and simmer about 10 more minutes over low heat.

2. Purée all the ingredients together in a food processor or blender. Serve hot or cold.

Per 2 Tbsp.: Calories: 20, Protein: 1 gm., Fat: 1 gm., Carbohydrates: 2 gm., Fiber: 6 gm., Sodium: 63 mg.

CURRIED CARROT SPREAD

YIELD: 1½ CUPS

Carrots contribute a colorful base for this mildly nippy spread.

½ lb. carrots, chopped
½ Tbsp. olive oil
1 medium onion, chopped
1 yellow bell pepper,
    chopped
2 cloves garlic, minced
2 tsp. curry powder
1 tsp. salt

1. Steam the carrots until soft.

2. Sauté the onion, yellow bell pepper, and garlic in the olive oil until transparent. Add the curry powder and salt, and cook another minute. Blend all the ingredients until smooth. Serve on fat-free crackers or bread, or use vegetables as dippers.

Per 2 Tbsp.: Calories: 19, Protein: 0 gm., Fat: 0 gm., Carbohydrates: 3 gm., Fiber: 1 gm., Sodium: 185 mg.

MINTED LENTIL SPREAD, PÂTÉ, OR DIP

YIELD: ABOUT 2 CUPS

A fresh twist on the trusty lentil.

2 cups cooked lentils
1 clove garlic, minced
¼ cup fresh mint,
    chopped
¼ cup green onion,
    chopped
1 Tbsp. soy sauce

1. Blend all the ingredients together in a food processor, chill, and serve.

Per 2 Tbsp.: Calories: 30, Protein: 2 gm., Fat: 0 gm., Carbohydrates: 5 gm., Fiber: 1 gm., Sodium: 63 mg.

TOFU-CILANTRO-GARLIC-JALAPEÑO DIP

YIELD: ABOUT 1½ CUPS

This makes a beautiful green, creamy, flavorful dip for chips or vegetables. Make it at least a few hours ahead of time so the flavors have time to blend. This also makes a great lower-fat, lower-calorie topping for burritos or tacos as a substitute for sour cream.

2 small cloves garlic
2 cups fresh cilantro leaves
1 small jalapeño, to taste
1-10.5 oz. pkg. lite silken tofu
2 Tbsp. fresh lime juice
½ tsp. salt (opt)

1. Chop the garlic, cilantro, and jalapeño in a food processor.

2. Add the tofu, lime juice, and salt, and blend until smooth. Chill and serve with baked tortilla chips or VEGETABLES FOR DIPPING (pg. 27).

Per 2 Tbsp.: Calories: 14, Protein: 2 gm., Fat: 0 gm., Carbohydrates: 1 gm., Fiber: 0 gm., Sodium: 25 mg.

CANNELLINI DIP OR SPREAD

YIELD: 1½ CUPS

This quick and easy spread offers a unique blend of Italian flavorings.

1¾ cups cooked cannellini
    beans, or 1-16 oz. can,
    drained
2 Tbsp. onion, chopped
1 large clove garlic, minced
½ tsp. fennel seed,
    crushed
½ tsp. basil
½ tsp. salt

1. Combine all the ingredients in a food processor, and blend until smooth. Refrigerate at least a few hours or overnight to let the flavors blend.

Per 2 Tbsp.: Calories: 31, Protein: 2 gm., Fat: 0 gm., Carbohydrates: 6 gm., Fiber: 1 gm., Sodium: 90 mg.

GARBANZO BEAN DIP (HUMMUS)

YIELD: 2 CUPS

Serve HUMMUS with wedges of pita bread or raw vegetables. It is tasty without the tahini or olive oil, which add another dimension of flavor but also more fat.

2 cloves garlic
¼ cup fresh parsley, packed
2 cups garbanzo beans
2 Tbsp. fresh lemon juice
1 Tbsp. tahini or olive oil (opt)
½ tsp. salt

1. Chop the garlic and parsley in a food processor or blender.

2. Add the rest of the ingredients, and blend until creamy.

Per 2 Tbsp.: Calories: 35, Protein: 2 gm., Fat: 0 gm., Carbohydrates: 6 gm., Fiber: 1 gm., Sodium: 69 mg.

GINGER-CINNAMON DIP FOR FRUIT

YIELD: ABOUT 1½ CUPS

This recipe calls for apples or pears, but any fruit in bite size pieces can be served. You might want to serve tooth picks with the stickier varieties of fruit. This can also be served as a topping for fruit, rather than as a dip.

1-10.5 oz. pkg. lite silken
   tofu
2 Tbsp. candied ginger,
   chopped
2 Tbsp. sweetener of choice
2 Tbsp. fresh lemon juice
¼ tsp. cinnamon
3 apples and/or pears,
   sliced
fresh lemon juice

1. Blend the tofu, ginger, sweetener, lemon juice, and cinnamon in a blender until smooth and creamy.

2. Cut the apples and/or pears into slices, and squirt with the fresh lemon juice to keep them from turning brown. Dip and enjoy.

Per ½ cup: Calories: 103, Protein: 4 gm., Fat: 1 gm., Carbohydrates: 20 gm., Fiber: 2 gm., Sodium: 57 mg.

Tofu-Miso Spread

Yield: 1½ cups

For the best flavor, this cheesy-tasting spread needs to be made ahead of time. Spread on crackers or bread, or use as a dip for chips or vegetables.

1 clove garlic
1-10.5 oz. pkg. lite silken
    tofu, or ½ lb reduced-fat
    firm tofu and 2 Tbsp.
    water
2 Tbsp. sweet rice miso
2 Tbsp. rice vinegar
2 tsp. onion powder

1. Chop the garlic in a food processor.

2. Add the rest of the ingredients, and blend until smooth. Refrigerate for a few hours or overnight for flavors to blend.

Per 2 Tbsp.: Calories: 17, Protein: 2 gm., Fat: 0 gm., Carbohydrates: 1 gm., Fiber: 0 gm., Sodium: 24 mg.

WHITE BEAN-HERB DIP OR SPREAD

These classic Italian gremolata flavorings are very quick and easy to put together. Roasted garlic gives a sweet, mild flavor.

2 cups cooked white beans,
   (cannellini, Great Northern, or navy), or
   1-15 oz. can, drained
2 cloves garlic, minced, or
   1 head roasted garlic
1 Tbsp. fresh lemon juice
½ tsp. fresh oregano
   leaves, minced
1 tsp. organic lemon zest
½ tsp. salt

1. Blend all the ingredients together in a food processor or blender until smooth.

2. Spread on crusty bread or serve with crackers or sweet pepper slices.

Per 2 Tbsp.: Calories: 32, Protein: 2 gm., Fat: 0 gm., Carbohydrates: 6 gm., Fiber: 1 gm., Sodium: 2 mg.

SALSAS

FRESH SWEET CORN SALSA

YIELD: 2½ CUPS

This is a unique way to enjoy fresh sweet corn. Make this salsa ahead of time to let the flavors blend.

2 cups fresh sweet corn, cut off the cob
½ cup sweet red bell pepper, chopped
½ cup fresh cilantro, loosely packed, then chopped
2 Tbsp. green onion, chopped
1 Tbsp. fresh lime juice
1 tsp. fresh jalapeño, minced
1 tsp. salt

1. Steam the fresh sweet corn for 3 minutes, cool, and cut off the cob.

2. Combine all the ingredients and refrigerate at least a few hours before serving.

Per 2 Tbsp.: Calories: 14, Protein: 0 gm., Fat: 0 gm., Carbohydrates: 3 gm., Fiber: 1 gm., Sodium: 110 mg.

CAPONATA

YIELD: 2 CUPS

This is a thick, rich eggplant relish that can be served on crackers, Italian bread, or lettuce as an appetizer or side dish.

1½ lbs. eggplant
2 heads garlic
1 Tbsp. olive oil
1 medium sweet onion, chopped
2 ribs celery, chopped
1 medium tomato, peeled and chopped
2 Tbsp. capers, chopped
2 Tbsp. raisins, chopped
2 Tbsp. wine vinegar
¼ cup black olives, chopped
¼ cup Italian parsley, chopped
¼ cup fresh basil, chopped
½ tsp. salt
⅛ tsp. cracked red pepper flakes
1 tsp. cocoa powder

1. Preheat the oven to 350°F.

2. Bake the eggplant (about one hour) and garlic (about 20 minutes) until soft. Peel and chop both.

3. Sauté the onion and celery in the olive oil until the onion is transparent. Stir in the rest of the ingredients, and simmer about 10 minutes. Cool and refrigerate if not serving right away. Serve at room temperature. Sprinkle with cocoa powder just before serving.

Per 2 Tbsp.: Calories: 37, Protein: 0 gm., Fat: 1 gm., Carbohydrates: 6 gm., Fiber: 1 gm., Sodium: 144 mg.

ROASTED PEPPER SALSA

YIELD: 2 CUPS

This combination of peppers gives a good flavor as well as a pleasing visual effect. You can use any combination of peppers to make it hot or mild or any combination of colors you like. Roasting the peppers adds a sweetness to the flavor and removes the tough skins.

1 sweet red bell pepper
1 sweet yellow bell pepper
1 sweet green pepper
1 jalapeño pepper (or to
    taste)

1. To roast the peppers, hold each one over an open flame or place under the broiler, turning until completely charred. Enclose the charred peppers in a paper or plastic bag to sweat for about 15 minutes, then peel, and remove the stems, membranes, and seeds from the peppers. If the pepper has been roasted long enough, the skins should come right off. You can peel them under running water. Remember, when peeling jalapeño peppers, wear disposable rubber gloves, and do not rub your eyes, nose, or any other mucous membrane.

2. Chop the peppers, mix, and serve as a salsa with raw vegetables, chips, or crackers or as an accompaniment to an entrée.

Per 2 Tbsp.: Calories: 4, Protein: 0 gm., Fat: 0 gm., Carbohydrates: 1 gm., Fiber: 0 gm., Sodium: 1 mg.

ITALIAN SALSA

YIELD: 2 CUPS

Try serving this tasty salsa with grilled tofu, tempeh, eggplant, zucchini, or Italian bread sticks.

1 lb. Roma tomatoes,
  peeled and chopped
  (about 1½ cups)
⅓ cup sweet fresh onion,
  chopped
⅓ cup fresh basil leaves,
  chopped
2 Tbsp. capers
1 Tbsp. kalamata olives,
  pitted and chopped (opt)
1 clove fresh garlic, crushed
1 Tbsp. red wine vinegar
2 tsp. strong olive oil (opt)

1. Mix all the ingredients together, and serve.

Per 2 Tbsp.: Calories: 7, Protein: 0 gm., Fat: 0 gm., Carbohydrates: 2 gm., Fiber: 0 gm., Sodium: 55 mg.

SALSA FRESCA

YIELD: 2 CUPS

Fresh salsa is a special treat. The best flavor is at the height of tomato and pepper season, when produce is plentiful and sweet. Canned tomatoes give a better flavor when tomatoes are out of season.

1 lb. plum tomatoes, peeled
   and chopped
½ cup fresh cilantro,
   chopped
½ cup sweet yellow
   onion, chopped
½-1 jalapeño, minced
1 clove garlic, pressed

1. Mix all the ingredients together. Serve with chips, raw vegetables, or any kind of Mexican entrée.

Per 2 Tbsp.: Calories: 8, Protein: 0 gm., Fat: 0 gm., Carbohydrates: 2 gm., Fiber: 0 gm., Sodium: 3 mg.

THAI SALSA

YIELD: 2 CUPS

Try serving as an accompaniment with BROILED TEMPEH OR TOFU *(pg. 112).*

2 cups cucumbers, peeled, seeded, and chopped
¼ cup green onions, chopped
½ cup fresh cilantro, chopped
1½ tsp. fresh ginger juice (pressed in a garlic press)
2 Tbsp. fresh lime juice
1 clove fresh garlic, pressed
½-1 fresh hot chili to taste, chopped

1. Mix all the ingredients together, and serve.

Per 2 Tbsp.: Calories: 7, Protein: 0 gm., Fat: 0 gm., Carbohydrates: 1 gm., Fiber: 1 gm., Sodium: 1 mg.

TOMATILLO-CHIPOTLE SALSA

YIELD: 1¼ CUPS

Chipotle pepper (smoked jalapéno pepper) adds a hot, smoky bite to this salsa, which is sometimes called "Salsa Verde" or Green Sauce.

1 lb. tomatillos
1 tsp. olive oil
1 small onion, chopped
½ tsp. dried, crushed
    chipotle pepper
½ cup fresh cilantro
    leaves, chopped

1. Remove the husks from the tomatillos, and chop.

2. Sauté the onion in the olive oil over low heat until transparent. Add the tomatillos and chipotle, and continue cooking until the tomatillos are soft. Turn off the heat and mix in the fresh cilantro leaves. Serve hot or cold.

Per 2 Tbsp.: Calories: 16, Protein: 0 gm., Fat: 0 gm., Carbohydrates: 2 gm., Fiber: 1 gm., Sodium: 4 mg.

Tropical Salsa

Yield: about 4 cups

Serve this tangy salsa with Broiled Tempeh or Tofu *(pg. 112) or crackers.*

1½ cups fresh mango, peeled, pitted, and chopped

1 cup fresh pineapple, peeled, cored, and chopped

1 cup sweet red bell pepper, chopped

½ cup sweet onion, chopped

¼ cup fresh cilantro, chopped

1 Tbsp. fresh lime juice

½ tsp. (or to taste) fresh hot pepper (serrano, jalapeño, or other)

1. Mix all the ingredients together up to 3 hours before serving.

Per 2 Tbsp.: Calories: 9, Protein: 0 gm., Fat: 0 gm., Carbohydrates: 2 gm., Fiber: 0 gm., Sodium: 2 mg.

FINGER FOODS

FRUIT KEBOBS

YIELD: 6 KEBOBS

Use any combination of fruits in season that appeals to you: melon balls, chunks of pineapple, whole berries, citrus sections, banana chunks, peaches, pears, papayas, mango, star fruit, etc.

3-4 cups fruit in season, cut in 1" chunks or balls
CREAMY SWEET-SOUR POPPY SEED DRESSING (pg. 45)

1. Prepare the fruit and skewer onto kebob sticks. Pour dressing over them, or serve the dressing on the side as a dip.

Per kebob: Calories: 142, Protein: 5 gm., Fat: 1 gm., Carbohydrates: 29 gm., Fiber: 1 gm., Sodium: 411 mg.

FROZEN GRAPES

YIELD: HOWEVER MANY YOU LIKE

For a crunchy change of pace, wash seedless grapes, pluck off the stem and freeze in a freezer bag. Serve as a frozen, crunchy, sweet treat.

Jícama Appetizer

This crispy tuber is a popular snack in markets in Mexico. Wait to sprinkle the dressing on until just at serving time, or it will become soggy.

½ lb. fresh jícama
½ fresh lime, squeezed
1 clove garlic, pressed
½ tsp. chili powder

1. Wash, peel, and cut the jícama into ¼" square sticks, like French fries.

2. Right before serving, sprinkle with the lime juice, garlic, and chili powder.

Per serving: Calories: 52, Protein: 1 gm., Fat: 0 gm., Carbohydrates: 12 gm., Fiber: 1 gm., Sodium: 3 mg.

VEGETABLES FOR DIPPING

YIELD: WHATEVER YOU LIKE

Almost any vegetable can be used as an accompaniment for dips and spreads. The smaller inner leaves of romaine or Boston lettuce make exceptionally nice dippers. Most vegetables can be served raw, but almost all of them can be enhanced by lightly steaming until the color intensifies and then plunging into ice water to stop the cooking process. This leaves the vegetables still crisp-tender and intensely colorful. The process also helps eliminate some of the gas associated with some raw vegetables. It can be done a few hours ahead of time, and the vegetables can then be refrigerated until time to serve. Try these with TOFU-CILANTRO-GARLIC-JALAPEÑO DIP *(pg. 11) or any of the salsas.*

SUGGESTED VEGETABLES FOR LIGHTLY STEAMING:
asparagus
broccoli
carrots
cauliflower
green, red, yellow, or any
**   other color bell pepper**
okra
parsnips
rutabagas
snow peas
string beans
zucchini or yellow summer
squash

1. Wash and cut the vegetables into desired shapes.

2. Steam only a minute or two until the color intensifies.

3. Plunge into ice water to cool down, and drain.

FRESH JUICES

I think the ultimate in non-fat, nutrient-packed snacks is fresh vegetable or fruit juice. Treat yourself and your family to your favorite combination of fruits and/or vegetables. If you don't have a juicer, consider investing in one for your health. Try to use only the freshest organic produce.

My favorite is fresh carrot juice. It takes about 1 pound of carrots to make 1 cup of juice. Sometimes I will add a small piece of gingerroot or an apple or a piece of lemon for variety. Sometimes I add fresh greens or celery. Try using the carrot pulp left from juicing in **BROILED OR GRILLED TOFU-CARROT BURGERS** (pg. 122) or **ORANGE CARROT SPICE CAKE** (pg. 147).

Remember that when you drink juice, you are not consuming the fibrous part of the vegetable, so juice is really not a replacement for eating vegetables. Be sure to take care if you have to watch your sugar intake. Most fresh juices are packed with natural sugars. Eating the whole fruit or vegetable in its natural form with all its fiber helps slow down the body's absorption of the sugars.

SALADS AND DRESSINGS

Salads can be a whole meal or an accent to a meal. Cooked beans, grains, tofu, tempeh, and pastas lend themselves well to salads that can make a whole meal, especially in the summertime.

I usually like to eat a generous salad made of a mixture of different kinds of lettuce, greens, and raw vegetables at the end of both my midday and evening meal. I grow or buy lettuce and raw vegetables of as many different varieties as possible, mixing different ones together to allow as much variety as I can. Raw foods still have their natural enzymes and vitamins which are destroyed by cooking. These enzymes aid digestion and promote health. Don't skimp on the mixed green salads; go ahead and enjoy your fill! Do go easy on the salad dressing if you use one with an oil base. Try using fresh lemon or lime juice for dressing or one of the tasty, lighter dressings included in this section.

SALADS AS A MAIN DISH

TEMPEH MACARONI SALAD

YIELD: 8 CUPS

This hearty pasta salad can be the center of a meal.

8 oz. tempeh
½ lb. shell or elbow
    macaroni
½ cup red bell pepper,
    chopped
1 cup celery, chopped
¼ cup green onions,
    chopped
½ cup sweet pickle
½ tsp. salt
¼ tsp. pepper
1-recipe ZIPPY TOFU SALAD
    DRESSING (pg. 43)

1. Steam the tempeh for 20 minutes, cool, and cube.

2. Cook the macaroni according to the package directions, rinse, and drain.

3. Toss all the ingredients together, and serve on a bed of green leaf lettuce.

Per cup: Calories: 124, Protein: 8 gm., Fat: 2 gm., Carbohydrates: 17 gm., Fiber: 2 gm., Sodium: 337 mg.

Taco Salad

This salad does well as a "build it yourself" salad with separate bowls of ingredients presented buffet style. This way each person can choose how much and what they want, and the salad doesn't get soggy. This makes a great summer buffet salad.

FOR EACH SERVING HAVE READY:

1 cup lettuce, various
varieties, torn

½ oz. baked corn tortilla
chips

½ cup cooked pinto beans
or black beans

¼ cup tomatoes, chopped
or sliced

¼ cup cucumber, chopped

2 Tbsp. avocado, chopped
and covered with a
squirt of lemon or lime

1 Tbsp. black olives, whole
or chopped

2 Tbsp. salsa, more or less
to taste

fresh cilantro, chopped

fresh lime or lemon wedges

1. Have each person arrange their salad in a large bowl like a pasta bowl or flat soup bowl in the order of ingredients listed here. Serve with SALSA FRESCA (pg. 21) or your favorite salsa and/or lime or lemon wedges as dressing. Top with optional TOFU-CILANTRO-GARLIC-JALAPEÑO DIP (pg. 11). Enjoy!

Per serving: Calories: 242, Protein: 8 gm., Fat: 7 gm., Carbohydrates: 35 gm., Fiber: 9 gm., Sodium: 374 mg.

QUINOA SALAD

YIELD: 5 CUPS

This colorful salad has a crunchy and chewy texture and a savory mixture of flavors, and features the ancient Incan staple, quinoa.

¾ cup quinoa
1½ cups boiling water
½ tsp. salt (opt)
1 cup carrots, grated
¼ lb. snow peas, sliced in
　¼" diagonals
¼ cup celery, chopped
¼ cup green onion,
　chopped
½ cup ZIPPY TOFU SALAD
　DRESSING (pg. 43)
　or reduced-fat tofu
　mayonnaise

1. Rinse the quinoa in a fine strainer, then stir into the boiling salted water. Cover and simmer over low heat for about 20 minutes. Fluff with a fork and cool.

2. Mix all the ingredients together, and serve.

Per cup: Calories: 126, Protein: 6 gm., Fat: 1 gm., Carbohydrates: 22 gm., Fiber: 4 gm., Sodium: 112 mg.

BLACK AND WHITE BEAN SALAD

YIELD: 4½ CUPS

This hearty and colorful blend can be a meal by itself.

1-15 oz. can black beans, drained

1-15 oz. can white beans, drained (Great Northern, navy, or cannellini)

½ cup sweet red pepper, finely chopped

½ cup sweet yellow pepper, finely chopped

½ cup green pepper, finely chopped

½ cup sweet red or yellow onions, finely chopped or green onions, finely chopped

¼ cup fresh cilantro, finely chopped

3 Tbsp. fresh lime juice

1 Tbsp. olive oil

½ tsp. salt

⅛ tsp. freshly ground black pepper

1. Mix the beans, peppers, onions, and cilantro together.

2. For the dressing, blend together the lime juice, olive oil, salt, and black pepper in a blender,.

3. Pour the dressing over the beans and vegetables, and mix well. Serve on a bed of lettuce garnished with fresh cilantro leaves.

Per cup: Calories: 300, Protein: 15 gm., Fat: 4 gm., Carbohydrates: 51 gm., Fiber: 10 gm., Sodium: 240 mg.

PASTA-GARBANZO SALAD

6 oz. small pasta spirals,
   shells, or ditalini pasta
   (2 cups cooked)
1-16 oz. can garbanzo
   beans, drained,
   or 2 cups cooked
   garbanzo beans
1 Tbsp. olive oil
1 Tbsp. lemon juice
1 Tbsp. balsamic vinegar
1 clove garlic, pressed
¼ cup fresh basil, loosely
   packed and chopped
1 sweet red bell pepper,
   chopped
¼ cup onion, chopped
½ lb. cherry tomatoes or
   roma tomatoes, peeled,
   seeded, and chopped
¼ lb. zucchini, chopped
   (uncooked)
½ tsp. salt
⅛ tsp. freshly ground black
   pepper

1. Cook the pasta in boiling water until tender, drain, and rinse.

2. Toss the pasta together with all the other ingredients, and serve.

Per cup: Calories: 158, Protein: 6 gm., Fat: 3 gm., Carbohydrates: 25 gm., Fiber: 4 gm., Sodium: 186 mg.

POTATO AND GREEN BEAN SALAD

YIELD: 4 CUPS

Here is a potato salad with Mediterranean flavors.

1 lb. new red potatoes
½ lb. young green beans,
  cut in 1" lengths,
  or 1-9 oz. pkg. frozen
  French cut green beans
1 Tbsp. olive oil
1 Tbsp. balsamic vinegar
½ tsp. salt
⅛ tsp. freshly ground black
  pepper
2 Tbsp. fresh parsley,
  chopped
2 tomatoes, cut in wedges

1. Steam the potatoes until tender, then peel and dice into ½" chunks.

2. Steam the green beans until tender.

3. While still hot, toss the potatoes and green beans together with the olive oil, vinegar, salt, black pepper, and parsley. Serve with tomato wedges.

Per cup: Calories: 147, Protein: 2 gm., Fat: 2 gm., Carbohydrates: 27 gm., Fiber: 4 gm., Sodium: 276 mg.

TABOULI SALAD

YIELD: 5 CUPS

This is a chewy, whole meal salad with Middle Eastern flavors.

½ cup bulgur wheat
1 cup boiling water
1 cup parsley, finely
   chopped
¼ cup fresh mint, finely
   chopped
¼ cup green onions,
   chopped
1 large tomato, diced
½ cucumber, peeled and
   diced
1 Tbsp. olive oil
2 Tbsp. fresh lemon juice
¼ tsp. salt
pinch of freshly ground
   black pepper
¼ cup black olives,
   chopped (opt)

1. Pour the boiling water over the bulgur wheat, and let stand for about one hour.

2. Drain and squeeze dry, then mix together with the rest of the ingredients. Toss all together and serve on a bed of lettuce garnished with mint leaves and tomato wedges.

Per cup: Calories: 110, Protein: 3 gm., Fat: 2 gm., Carbohydrates: 18 gm., Fiber: 3 gm., Sodium: 117 mg.

Light Salads

Thai Slaw

YIELD: 6 CUPS (6-8 SERVINGS)

This colorful slaw with a new taste twist is pictured on the cover.

FOR THE *DRESSING:*
1 clove garlic, crushed
1 Tbsp. gingerroot, minced
2 Tbsp. sweetener of choice
1 Tbsp. toasted sesame oil
3 Tbsp. fresh lemon juice
2 Tbsp. water
¼ cup dry roasted peanuts
½ tsp. jalapeño, or ¼ tsp.
   cracked red pepper

FOR THE *SLAW:*
4 cups cabbage, finely
   shredded (¾ lb.)
1 cup cucumber, seeded
   and chopped
¼ cup green onion
½ red bell pepper, sliced
1 cup fresh cilantro, loosely
   packed and chopped

1. Prepare the *DRESSING:* Chop all the ingredients for the dressing in order in a food processor until blended.

2. Prepare the *SLAW:* Cut the slaw vegetables, toss together with the dressing, and serve.

Per serving: Calories: 85, Protein: 2 gm., Fat: 4 gm., Carbohydrates: 10 gm., Fiber: 2 gm., Sodium: 13 mg.

CARROT-RUTABAGA-TURNIP SLAW

YIELD: 4 CUPS

A colorful range of golds to oranges with flecks of green tempt the eye to this flavorful slaw.

1 medium rutabaga, peeled
and grated (about 2 cups)
1 medium turnip, peeled
and grated (about 1 cup)
1 cup carrots, grated
1 Tbsp. onion, finely grated
2 Tbsp. fresh lemon juice
2 Tbsp. fresh mint, chopped
2 tsp. olive oil
½ tsp. salt
⅛ tsp. freshly ground
black pepper

1. Toss all the ingredients together, and serve, or refrigerate and let the flavors blend overnight.

Per cup: Calories: 71, Protein: 1 gm., Fat: 2 gm., Carbohydrates: 11 gm., Fiber: 3 gm., Sodium: 311 mg.

Beet Salad
with Orange Vinaigrette

Yield: 6 servings

Here is the humble but nutritious beet dressed in a fruity, sweet-sour dressing.

1 lb. baby beets or large
   beets, cut in small chunks
¼ cup orange juice
2 Tbsp. apple cider vinegar
2 Tbsp. organic orange zest,
   freshly grated
½ Tbsp. olive oil
½ tsp. salt
3 Tbsp. sweet onion,
   minced
1 small orange, peeled and
   sectioned

1. Wash and trim the beets, then steam until tender.

2. Blend the orange juice, vinegar, orange zest, olive oil, and salt in a blender. Pour over the hot, steamed beets, and toss together with the onion and orange sections. Refrigerate overnight before serving to let the flavors blend. Serve on a bed of Boston lettuce leaves.

Per serving: Calories: 41, Protein: 1 gm., Fat: 1 gm., Carbohydrates: 7 gm., Fiber: 2 gm., Sodium: 215 mg.

Tomato Vegetable Aspic

YIELD: 4-6 SERVINGS

Kanten is a dried flake gelatin made from sea weed and is available in natural food stores.

2 cups tomato-vegetable juice cocktail

1 Tbsp. fresh lime or lemon juice

3 Tbsp. kanten flakes

¼ cup green onion, chopped

¼ cup celery, chopped

¼ cup sweet yellow or green pepper, chopped

¼ cup cucumber, seeded and chopped

½ avocado, chopped

1. Mix the juices and kanten flakes together, and let soften for 15 minutes. *Microwave Method:* Heat the mixture on high power for 6 minutes, stopping and stirring at 3 minutes. All the kanten should be dissolved. *Stovetop Method:* Bring the mixture to a boil in a saucepan, reduce heat, and simmer 5 minutes.

2. Stir in the green onion, celery, sweet yellow pepper, cucumber, and avocado, and pour into a single mold or individual molds, which have first been rinsed with cold water. Chill until firm. To release the salad from the mold, first set the mold in very hot water for a few minutes, then invert it on to a bed of lettuce.

Per serving: Calories: 63, Protein: 2 gm., Fat: 2 gm., Carbohydrates: 8 gm., Fiber: 2 gm., Sodium: 27 mg.

STRAWBERRY GEL

YIELD: 2 CUPS (4 SERVINGS)

This can be served as a salad or dessert. Make it with or without chunks of added fruit. Kanten is a dried flake gelatin made from sea weed and is available in natural food stores.

3½-4 cups strawberries, to make 2 cups purée
2 Tbsp. sweetener of choice, or to taste
2 Tbsp. kanten flakes
1-2 cups fresh fruit of choice, cut in chunks (opt)

1. Blend the strawberries in a blender or food processor until liquefied. Stir the kanten into the blended berries. *Stovetop Method:* Bring the berries and kanten to a boil, reduce the heat, and simmer 5 minutes. *Microwave Method:* Heat the berries and kanten until boiling, then microwave 5 more minutes.

2. Pour the liquid into a 6 cup mold, and chill until firm. If you are adding the optional chunks of fruit, arrange them in the mold before pouring in the liquid.

Per serving: Calories: 65, Protein: 1 gm., Fat: 0 gm., Carbohydrates: 15 gm., Fiber: 3 gm., Sodium: 2 mg.

MIXED GREEN SALAD

YIELD: AS MUCH AS YOU LIKE

A green salad compliments so many different main dishes; it is one the most versatile and low calorie dishes to serve. A salad that is the equivalent of ¼ head of lettuce contains about 17 calories and only a trace of fat. Always pleasing to the eye, a mixed green salad can be as simple or complex as you like. Try different combinations of the many different types of salad greens available. Don't be limited to iceberg lettuce; use romaine, butter, Boston, red leaf, green leaf, arugula, escarole, spinach, red cabbage, green cabbage, mixtures of baby gourmet lettuce (mesclun), or whatever looks good to you.

Add some color accent to the greens by cutting up red, yellow, orange, or purple bell peppers. Grate or slice some carrot, and cut up a cucumber or some radishes. Cut up a tomato or add cherry tomatoes. Add purple or sweet yellow onion, or chop up some green onion. Add raw broccoli or cauliflower florets, or toss in some sunflower sprouts. The list goes on and on. Just use your imagination and the freshest ingredients you can find.

My favorite dressing for salad is a squeeze of fresh lemon or lime juice, which adds zing and flavor but no fat. There are a number of fat-free salad dressings on the market that you could try if you are so inclined. Try a bit of **CILANTRO-WALNUT PESTO** (pg. 48), **FRESH HERB DRESSING** (pg. 47), or **LIGHT TOFU-MISO DRESSING** (pg. 46) tossed into the salad. I usually serve salad without dressing, and let each individual decide how to dress it.

Salad Dressings, Sauces, and Pestos

Zippy Tofu Salad Dressing

YIELD: 1½ CUPS

This is a replacement for mayonnaise that has no added fat. It has a zippy bite to it that adds a zing to sandwiches and salads. It will keep in the refrigerator for about a week.

1-10.5 oz. pkg. lite silken tofu
2 Tbsp. apple cider vinegar
1 Tbsp. sweetener of your choice
½ tsp. salt
⅛ tsp. dry mustard
¼ tsp. garlic powder

1. Blend all the ingredients together in a blender or food processor until smooth and creamy.

Per Tbsp.: Calories: 8, Protein: 1 gm., Fat: 0 gm., Carbohydrates: 1 gm., Fiber: 0 gm., Sodium: 56 mg.

CREAMY BASIL DRESSING OR SAUCE

YIELD: ABOUT 1½ CUPS

This sauce is equally yummy hot over pasta or chilled as a salad dressing.

1 clove garlic
2 cups fresh basil leaves,
  loosely packed
1–10.5 oz. pkg. lite silken
  tofu
½ tsp. salt

1. Chop the garlic and basil in a food processor. Add the tofu and salt, and process until creamy.

2. Serve cold or hot. If serving hot, heat but do not boil.

Per Tbsp.: Calories: 8, Protein: 1 gm., Fat: 0 gm., Carbohydrates: 1 gm., Fiber: 0 gm., Sodium: 56 mg.

LIGHT TOFU SOUR CREAM

YIELD: 1½ CUPS

This dressing has no added fat and no cholesterol and can be served anytime you would serve sour cream. You can vary the flavor by adding small amounts of different herbs or spices, depending on what you are serving with it.

1–10.5 oz. pkg. lite silken
  tofu
1½ Tbsp. fresh lemon juice
2 tsp. sweetener of your
  choice
½ tsp. salt

1. Blend all the ingredients together in a blender or food processor until smooth and creamy.

Per Tbsp.: Calories: 7, Protein: 1 gm., Fat: 0 gm., Carbohydrates: 1 gm., Fiber: 0 gm., Sodium: 12 mg.

CREAMY SWEET-SOUR POPPY SEED DRESSING

YIELD: ABOUT 2 CUPS

Use this pungent, sweet-sour dressing for fruit salad or as a dip for **Fruit Kebobs** *(pg. 25).*

1-10.5 oz. pkg. lite silken
   tofu
½ cup apple cider vinegar
⅓ cup honey or sweetener
   of your choice
2 Tbsp. onion, minced
2 Tbsp. poppy seeds
1½ tsp. dry mustard
1 tsp. salt
1 tsp. paprika

1. Blend all the ingredients in a blender or food processor until smooth and creamy.

Per Tbsp.: Calories: 16, Protein: 1 gm., Fat: 0 gm., Carbohydrates: 3 gm., Fiber: 0 gm., Sodium: 76 mg.

HONEY-MUSTARD DRESSING OR DIP

YIELD: ½ CUP

Use as a dressing for salads or steamed vegetables or as a dip for ARTICHOKES (pg. 130).

¼ cup Dijon or natural stone ground mustard
2 Tbsp. honey
2 Tbsp. cider vinegar
1 Tbsp. olive oil (opt)

1. Blend all the ingredients together in a blender or food processor until smooth and creamy.

Per Tbsp.: Calories: 19, Protein: 0 gm., Fat: 0 gm., Carbohydrates: 3 gm., Fiber: 1 gm., Sodium: 90 mg.

LIGHT TOFU-MISO DRESSING

YIELD: ABOUT 1¾ CUP

1-10.5 oz. pkg. lite silken tofu
4 Tbsp. apple cider or rice vinegar
4 Tbsp. sweet white miso
2 tsp. sweetener of your choice
½ tsp. garlic powder
¼ tsp. freshly ground black pepper

1. Blend all the ingredients together in a blender or food processor until smooth and creamy.

Per Tbsp.: Calories: 18, Protein: 1 gm., Fat: 1 gm., Carbohydrates: 1 gm., Fiber: 0 gm., Sodium: 1 mg.

Fresh Herb Dressings

Perk up your salad with these fresh herb dressings.

Fresh Basil-Parsley-Garlic Dressing

YIELD: 6 TBSP.

2 cloves garlic
½ oz. fresh basil
¼ oz. fresh Italian parsley
2 Tbsp. balsamic vinegar
1 Tbsp. olive oil (opt)

1. Chop the garlic, basil, and parsley in a food processor or blender.

2. Blend in the vinegar and oil.

Per Tbsp.: Calories: 24, Protein: 0 gm., Fat: 2 gm., Carbohydrates: 1 gm., Fiber: 0 gm., Sodium: 1 mg.

Fresh Arugula-Parsley-Garlic Dressing

YIELD: 6 TBSP.

2 cloves garlic
½ oz. fresh arugula
¼ oz. fresh parsley
2 Tbsp. balsamic vinegar
1 Tbsp. olive oil (opt)

1. Chop the garlic, arugula, and parsley in a food processor or blender.

2. Blend in the vinegar and oil.

Per Tbsp.: Calories: 24, Protein: 0 gm., Fat: 2 gm., Carbohydrates: 1 gm., Fiber: 0 gm., Sodium: 1 mg.

PESTOS

These flavorful pestos are delicious as a salad dressing or as a topping for steamed vegetables, grains, or pasta to replace butter or margarine. They can be stored in the freezer for a few months. For individual servings, drop the pesto by tablespoon into ice cube trays and freeze. When frozen, remove the cubes from the trays, and store in a freezer bag.

CILANTRO-WALNUT PESTO

YIELD: 6 TBSP.

4 cups cilantro leaves, loosely packed
¼ cup walnuts
1½ Tbsp. fresh lemon juice
¼ tsp. salt

1. Chop the cilantro leaves in a food processor. Add the walnuts and chop until blended. Add the lemon juice and salt, and blend again. Toss into salad as a salad dressing, or mix into pasta, steamed vegetables, or grains.

Per Tbsp.: Calories: 36, Protein: 1 gm., Fat: 3 gm., Carbohydrates: 2 gm., Fiber: 0 gm., Sodium: 92 mg.

BASIL-PIGNOLI PESTO

YIELD: 8 TBSP.

4 cups fresh basil leaves, loosely packed
4 cloves garlic
½ tsp. salt
¼ cup pignoli (pine nuts)

1. Blend all the ingredients together in a food processor or blender until smooth.

Per Tbsp.: Calories: 38, Protein: 2 gm., Fat: 2 gm., Carbohydrates: 3 gm., Fiber: 2 gm., Sodium: 146 mg.

SOUPS

There is nothing more appealing on a cold winter's day than a steaming hot, hearty bowl of soup. And conversely, chilled soup on a hot summer's day can really hit the spot. Each season offers its' own special produce to add an endless variety of flavors and textures to your soup pot. Hearty or light, steaming or chilled, soup is always a welcome sight on the table.

Main Dish Soups

Minted Lentil Soup

Yield: 3 cups

A hint of mint gives a new twist to lentil soup.

1½ cups cooked lentils
1½ cups water
1 Tbsp. fresh mint, chopped
1 clove garlic, minced
¼ cup green onions or
    sweet onions, chopped
½ tsp. salt
⅛ tsp. freshly ground black
    pepper

1. Simmer all the ingredients together until the onions are tender.

2. Blend in a food processor or blender until smooth. Serve hot.

Per cup: Calories: 117, Protein: 8 gm., Fat: 0 gm., Carbohydrates: 21 gm., Fiber: 3 gm, Sodium: 358 mg.

Savory White Kidney Bean Soup or Sauce for Pasta

Yield: 5 cups

Here's a meal that is quick and easy to prepare. You can serve it as a soup with crusty bread and vegies or as a sauce for pasta.

2 tsp. olive oil
1 large onion, chopped
    (1 cup)
1 sweet yellow pepper,
    chopped (1 cup)
2 cloves garlic, minced
1 carrot, sliced (½ cup)
½ cup celery, sliced
2 cups water
1-16 oz. can white kidney
    or cannellini beans,
    drained, or 2 cups
    cooked beans
½ tsp. salt
½ tsp. sage
¼ tsp. rosemary
¼ tsp. thyme
⅛ tsp. freshly ground black
    pepper
½ cup fresh parsley,
    chopped

1. In a soup pot, briefly sauté the onion, yellow pepper, garlic, carrot, and celery in the olive oil. Add the water, beans, salt, sage, rosemary, thyme, and black pepper. Simmer about 8 minutes or until the vegetables are tender. Add the parsley, and simmer 2 more minutes. Serve hot as a soup or over pasta.

Per cup: Calories: 143, Protein: 7 gm., Fat: 1 gm., Carbohydrates: 24 gm., Fiber: 5 gm, Sodium: 246 mg.

SUCCOTASH SOUP

YIELD: 6 CUPS

A quick and easy variation on a southern classic.

3 cups water
2 cups canned or frozen
   lima beans
2 cups fresh or frozen corn
   kernels
½ cup onion, chopped
½ cup green pepper,
   chopped
½ cup celery, chopped
¼ cup parsley, chopped
2 cloves garlic, pressed
1 tsp. salt
1 tsp. marjoram or oregano
½ tsp. thyme
⅛ tsp. freshly ground black
   pepper

1. Combine all the ingredients in a soup pot, heat thoroughly, and simmer together for about 10 minutes. Serve hot.

Per cup: Calories: 118, Protein: 5 gm., Fat: 0 gm., Carbohydrates: 24 gm., Fiber: 7 gm, Sodium: 389 mg.

CHICK-PEA NOODLE SOUP

YIELD: ABOUT 6 CUPS

This is a quick vegetarian version of the renowned "chicken soup."

1 cup cooked chick-peas
½ cup water
1 Tbsp. onion powder
1 tsp. garlic powder
5 cups water
2 Tbsp. low sodium soy
    sauce
2 Tbsp. nutritional yeast
    (opt)
¼ tsp. freshly ground black
    pepper
¼ lb. flat noodles
1 bay leaf
¼ cup fresh parsley,
    chopped

1. Purée the chick-peas, ½ cup water, onion powder, and garlic powder in a blender.

2. Bring the 5 cups water to a boil in a soup pot, and add the chick-pea purée, soy sauce, nutritional yeast, and black pepper. Bring to a boil again, and add the noodles and bay leaf. Boil until the pasta is almost tender, then stir in the parsley. Simmer until the pasta is tender, and serve.

Per cup: Calories 70, Protein 3 gm., Fat 0 gm., Carbohydrates 13 gm., Fiber 2 gm, Sodium 203 mg.

VARIATION: CHICK-PEA NOODLE VEGETABLE SOUP: Along with the noodles, add 1 large carrot, cut into match-stick pieces and ⅔ cup green peas (fresh or frozen), or ⅔ cup green onions, chopped, including the greens.

Per cup: Calories: 89, Protein: 4 gm., Fat: 0 gm., Carbohydrates: 16 gm., Fiber: 3 gm, Sodium: 209 mg.

FAGIOLI

YIELD: ABOUT 8 CUPS

This is a delightful Italian vegetable soup. The quickest way to make this soup is to start with canned beans. (You can also pressure cook ¾ cup dried beans or slow cook them overnight.) The actual preparation of the vegetables takes only a few minutes. You can substitute any kind of white beans for cannellini.

3 cups water
½ cup carrots, thinly sliced
1 medium onion, chopped
1-16 oz. can cannellini beans, or ¾ cup dried
1-16 oz. can diced tomatoes, or 1¾ cups plum tomatoes, chopped
1 cup green beans, cut in 1" pieces
½ lb. zucchini, sliced
1 clove garlic, crushed
½ cup celery, sliced
½ red bell pepper, chopped
½ yellow bell pepper, chopped
½ cup ditalini pasta
¼ cup parsley, chopped
¼ cup fresh basil, chopped
1 tsp. salt
¼ tsp. freshly ground black pepper

1. ***Open Kettle Method using canned beans:*** Bring the water to a boil in a soup kettle, add the carrots and onion, and simmer until almost tender. Add the rest of the ingredients, bring to a boil again, and simmer until all the vegetables are tender. ***Pressure Cooker Method using dried beans:*** Cook ¾ cup dried white kidney or Great Northern beans until tender in a pressure cooker. (Soaked beans take about 15 minutes, unsoaked about 25 minutes.) Bring the pressure down, open the cooker, and add the tomatoes, green beans, zucchini, carrots, onion, garlic, celery, bell peppers, and ditalini. Close the pressure cooker, bring back to pressure, and cook for 5 minutes. Immediately cool down the pressure cooker, and add the rest of the ingredients. Simmer together for a few minutes, and serve.

Per cup: Calories: 142, Protein: 7 gm., Fat: 0 gm., Carbohydrates: 28 gm., Fiber: 6 gm, Sodium: 294 mg.

PINTO AND TORTILLA SOUP

YIELD: 4½ CUPS

This is a simple but delicious, mildly picante soup.

1-10 oz. can tomatoes and green chilies
20 oz. water (2 cans)
1-16 oz. can pinto beans, drained
1 cup fresh cilantro, chopped
4 tortillas cut in thin slices
½ avocado
fresh cilantro leaves

1. Combine the tomatoes, green chilies, water, pinto beans, and cilantro in a saucepan or microwave-safe bowl, and heat to a simmer.

2. Heat the tortillas on a non-stick griddle, only briefly until soft. Cut into thin strips.

3. Cut the avocado into thin strips.

4. Ladle the steaming soup into bowls, and top with tortilla strips. Arrange the avocado strips and cilantro leaves on top, and serve.

Per cup: Calories: 256, Protein: 10 gm., Fat: 5 gm., Carbohydrates: 42 gm., Fiber: 7 gm, Sodium: 107 mg.

CHIPOTLE SPLIT PEA SOUP

YIELD: ABOUT 10 CUPS

Chipotle is a smoked jalapeño pepper that gives a smoky flavor without the ham hock.

2 cups dried split peas
8 cups boiling water
1 medium onion, chopped
2 cloves garlic, minced
2 carrots, sliced diagonally
2 stalks celery, sliced
   diagonally
½ cup parsley, chopped
½ chipotle, finely cut (1
   tsp.) or more to taste
1 Tbsp. low-sodium soy
   sauce

1. Simmer the split peas in boiling water until soft, about 1 hour.

2. Add the onion, garlic, carrots, celery, parsley, chipotle, and soy sauce. Continue cooking until the vegetables are tender, adding more water as needed.

Per cup: Calories: 107, Protein: 6 gm., Fat: 0 gm., Carbohydrates: 20 gm., Fiber: 5 gm, Sodium: 105 mg.

GREAT NORTHERN VEGETABLE SOUP

YIELD: ABOUT 10 CUPS

This quick, hearty, steaming hot soup will warm up a cold winters day.

8 cups water
4 oz. tomato paste
2 cups cooked Great
    Northern beans, or 1-16
    oz. can, drained
1 medium onion, chopped
1 clove garlic, minced
1 large carrot, sliced
1 medium potato, cut in
    ¼" cubes (about 1 cup)
1 cup green beans, chopped
1 cup sweet corn
1 cup green peas
1 tsp. salt
1 bay leaf
½ tsp. oregano
½ tsp. basil
¼ tsp. black pepper
½ cup fresh parsley,
    chopped

1. Bring the water to a boil in a soup pot, and stir in the tomato paste. Add the rest of the ingredients, except the parsley, and simmer until the vegetables are tender. Add more water for a thinner soup, and salt to taste. Stir in the parsley just before serving.

Per cup: Calories: 109, Protein: 4 gm., Fat: 0 gm., Carbohydrates: 22 gm., Fiber: 5 gm, Sodium: 236 mg.

Sopa de Frijoles Negros
(Black Bean Soup)

YIELD: ABOUT 9 CUPS

You can cook up a large pot of this soup and freeze individual servings for quick meals later on. Long, slow cooking is the preferred method for full-flavor, but the quick bean cooking methods make a tasty soup as well.

2 cups dried black beans
4 cloves garlic, minced
1 bay leaf
8 cups water
1 large onion, chopped
1 poblano or green pepper,
   chopped
2 tsp. salt
½ cup fresh cilantro leaves,
   chopped

1. Cook the black beans, garlic, and bay leaf in the water until the beans are tender. (Pressure cook unsoaked beans 90 minutes, soaked beans 45 minutes. In an open kettle, cook unsoaked beans about 6 hours, soaked beans 3 hours.)

2. Add the onion, poblano pepper, and salt to the pot. Simmer until the vegetables are almost tender, then stir in the cilantro. Simmer a few more minutes, and serve.

Per cup: Calories: 136, Protein: 7 gm., Fat: 0 gm., Carbohydrates: 25 gm., Fiber: 5 gm, Sodium: 476 mg.

VARIATIONS: *TO START WITH COOKED OR CANNED BEANS:* Use 6 cups of cooked beans or 3–16 oz. cans. Add enough water to make 8 cups in all. Heat to simmering and add the rest of the ingredients. Simmer until the vegetables are tender and serve.

TO START WITH INSTANT DEHYDRATED BEANS: Reconstitute the beans according to package directions to equal 6 cups hydrated beans, then add enough water to make 8 cups in all. Heat to simmering and add the rest of the ingredients. Simmer until the vegetables are tender, and serve.

LIGHT SOUPS

WATERCRESS SOUP

YIELD: 5 CUPS

This light and creamy soup can be served hot in cold weather or cold in hot weather. It has an alluring bright green color.

1 tsp. olive or canola oil

1 large onion, chopped, or
    4 leeks (white part only),
    chopped

2 large cloves garlic, minced

4 cups water

1 lb. russet potatoes, peeled
    and chopped

4 cups watercress leaves,
    washed, trimmed, and
    packed

½–10.5 oz. pkg. lite silken
    tofu

1 tsp. salt

⅛ tsp. freshly ground black
    pepper

1. In a soup pot, sauté the onion and garlic in the oil until tender. Add the water to the pot, and bring to a boil. Add the potatoes and simmer until soft (about 15 minutes). Add the watercress and continue to simmer for 3 to 4 minutes or just until the leaves start to wilt.

2. Pour into a food processor along with the tofu, salt, and black pepper. Process until smooth and creamy. If you are serving the soup hot, pour back into the soup pot, and heat to a simmer (do not boil). If you are serving the soup cold, transfer to a container, and refrigerate until thoroughly chilled. Serve with a fresh sprig of watercress or an edible flower floating on top.

Per cup: Calories: 112, Protein: 4 gm., Fat: 2 gm., Carbohydrates: 21 gm., Fiber: 3 gm, Sodium: 471 mg.

MUSHROOM BARLEY SOUP

YIELD: 5 CUPS

This is a very delicately flavored, easy-to-digest soup.

1 tsp. sesame oil
½ cup barley, rinsed and
    drained
4 cups boiling water or
    soup stock
1 large carrot, cut in match
    sticks or slices
½ cup green onions,
    chopped
8 oz. mushrooms, sliced
1 Tbsp. low-sodium soy
    sauce

1. In a soup pot, toast the barley in the sesame oil until lightly browned (about 7 to 10 minutes). Add the boiling water to the pot, and simmer, covered, for about 25 minutes.

2. Stir in the carrot, green onions, mushrooms, and soy sauce, and simmer until the carrots are tender. Add a little water if necessary to keep the vegetables covered with broth. Salt to taste and serve.

Per cup: Calories: 131, Protein: 2 gm., Fat: 0 gm., Carbohydrates: 11 gm., Fiber: 2 gm, Sodium: 131 mg.

BORSCHT

YIELD: 4½ CUPS

This soup is delicious hot or cold. Do your grating in the food processor to save time.

3 cups water
2 cups beets, grated
1 cup carrots, grated
1 cup tomatoes, diced
⅓ cup onions, minced
1 bay leaf
2 cups beet greens and/or
   cabbage, shredded
2 Tbsp. fresh lemon juice
1 Tbsp. sweetener of choice
½ tsp. salt
⅛ tsp. freshly ground black
   pepper

1. Bring the water to a boil, then add the beets, carrots, tomatoes, onions, and bay leaf. Simmer for about 5 minutes or until the vegetables are tender.

2. Add the greens, lemon juice, sweetener, salt, and black pepper. Simmer about 5 more minutes or until the greens are tender. Serve hot or cold.

Per cup: Calories: 82, Protein: 1 gm., Fat: 0 gm., Carbohydrates: 19 gm., Fiber: 4 gm, Sodium: 291 mg.

FRESH SWEET PEA SOUP

YIELD: 3½ CUPS

Try this fresh taste of spring for a light meal.

1 tsp. sesame oil

2 leeks (white part only),
  chopped, or ¾ cup
  sweet onion, chopped

2 cups boiling water

3 cups fresh or frozen sweet
  green peas, shelled

3 cups Bibb, romaine, or
  Boston lettuce, chopped

2 Tbsp. fresh mint leaves,
  chopped

½ tsp. salt

⅛ tsp. freshly ground black
  pepper

1. Sauté the leeks in the sesame oil over low heat until soft. Add the boiling water, peas, and lettuce. Bring to a boil and simmer about 10 minutes.

2. Stir in the mint, salt, and black pepper. Purée in a food processor or blender, and serve hot with a dollop of LIGHT TOFU SOUR CREAM (pg. 44).

Per cup: Calories: 311, Protein: 7 gm., Fat: 2 gm., Carbohydrates: 25 gm., Fiber: 7 gm, Sodium: 311 mg.

MISO SOUP

YIELD: ABOUT 8 CUPS (SERVES 6-8)

Miso is a salty, cultured paste made from soybeans or grains. It makes a wonderful soup base. The darker varieties tend to have a stronger flavor than the lighter ones. Don't ever let it boil, or it will become cloudy and separate.

6 cups water
1 carrot, cut in match stick size pieces
1 small onion, cut in rounds
½ lb. watercress or spinach, coarsely chopped
½ cup sweet white miso

1. Bring the water to a boil, and add the carrot. Simmer until tender. Turn off the heat and add the onion and watercress.

2. Dip out ½ cup hot water from the pot, and mix together with the miso. Stir until the miso mixture is smooth, then pour it back into the soup pot, and stir. Do not boil. Serve immediately.

Per cup: Calories: 57, Protein: 3 gm., Fat: 1 gm., Carbohydrates: 8 gm., Fiber: 3 gm, Sodium: 31 mg.

VARIATION: You can add ¼ lb. reduced-fat tofu or ½ package lite silken tofu cut in small cubes to the soup along with the onions and watercress.

Per cup: Calories 70, Protein 5 gm., Fat 1 gm., Carbohydrates 9 gm., Fiber 3 gm, Sodium 61 mg.

CHUNKY GAZPACHO

This is best in the summer made with fresh vine ripened tomatoes.

2 Tbsp. sweet onion
2 cloves garlic
2 lbs. fresh, ripe tomatoes, peeled (2½-3 cups)
1 large cucumber, peeled, seeded, and coarsely chopped (2 cups)
1 green bell pepper, seeded
½ cup fresh parsley or fresh basil
2 Tbsp. red wine vinegar
½ tsp. salt
tomato juice (opt)

1. Mince the onion and garlic in a food processor. Add the tomatoes, cucumber, bell pepper, parsley, vinegar, and salt to the processor, and chop only until chunky.

2. If the soup is too thick, add the optional tomato juice. Serve with an optional dollop of LIGHT TOFU SOUR CREAM (pg. 44) and a sprinkle of chives.

Per cup: Calories: 66, Protein: 2 gm., Fat: 0 gm., Carbohydrates: 13 gm., Fiber: 5 gm, Sodium: 291 mg.

MAINLY BEANS

Versatile beans are power-packed with protein, iron, and calcium. They are a good source of dietary fiber, vitamins, and minerals and come in a wide variety of flavors, colors, and textures. One half cup of cooked beans contains 5 to 10 grams of protein, 6 to 9 grams of fiber, and less than 1 gram of fat. (The exceptions are soybeans with about 5 grams of fat and chick-peas with about 2 grams of fat per half cup.)

I keep beans stocked in several forms in the pantry: dried beans in sealed, air tight containers, canned beans, and dehydrated instant beans. Check the labels on canned and dehydrated instant beans to make sure they have no added fat.

There are several different basic cooking methods for beans. Soaking the beans in water overnight always shortens the cooking time. To quick soak dried beans: Place the beans in a cooking pot, pour boiling water over them, return the pot to a boil, turn off the heat, and let them soak for 10 to 15 minutes. Drain, rinse, cover with fresh water, and cook. Long, slow cooking usually results in the most flavorful beans. Either a slow cooker or crock pot works well, and you can cook while you are out of the kitchen! An open pot on the stovetop will do the job as well, but you must make sure the beans are always covered with water. A pressure cooker is a fuel and time saver for cooking beans. It will cook soaked or unsoaked beans.

Canned beans and dehydrated instant beans are fast foods. A 16 oz. can of beans yields about 1¾ cups of beans that are ready to eat. Add boiling water to dehydrated instant beans, let them set 5 minutes, and they are ready to eat.

There are hundreds of different varieties of beans to choose from including: adzuki (aduki, azuki), anasazi, black turtle, garbanzo (chick-peas), cranberry, fava, lentil (many different types), lima, mung, pinto, small red, red kidney, white kidney (cannellini), Great Northern, navy, soy, and more.

CHICK-PEA AND TOMATO CURRY

YIELD: 4 CUPS

This is a quick and easy curry to be served over rice.

2 tsp. canola oil
½ tsp. curry powder
¼ tsp. cumin
¼ tsp. cinnamon
¼ tsp. black pepper
1 bay leaf
1 square inch fresh gingerroot
1 cup onions, chopped
3 cloves garlic, crushed
3 cups tomatoes, peeled and
   chopped
2 cups cooked chick-peas,
   or 1-16 oz. can

1. Gently bubble the spices, except the gingerroot, in the canola oil over low heat.

2. Peel the ginger and crush it in a garlic press, saving the juice for the curry and discarding the fiber. Add the onions, garlic, and ginger juice, and sauté until the onions are soft. Add the tomatoes and chick-peas, and simmer all together about 10 minutes to meld flavors. Serve over rice.

Per 2 Tbsp.: Calories: 26, Protein: 1 gm., Fat: 0 gm., Carbohydrates: 4 gm., Fiber 1 gm., Sodium: 3 mg.

LOUISIANA RED BEANS AND RICE

YIELD: 4½ CUPS

The cooking time will vary depending on the method used to cook the beans. Canned beans can be used, but the best flavor comes from long, slow cooking. Use a slow cooker or crockpot if you have one.

1 cup dried red kidney
    beans, or 1-16 oz. can
about 6 cups water
1 large onion, chopped
1 green pepper, chopped
2 stalks celery, chopped
1 clove garlic, minced,
    or ½ tsp. garlic powder
½ cup parsley, chopped,
    or 2 Tbsp. dry parsley
1 bay leaf
1 tsp. salt
1/2 tsp. thyme
1/2 tsp. oregano
1/4 tsp. freshly ground
    black pepper
1/8 tsp. dry mustard
1/8 tsp. cayenne pepper
1 Tbsp. oil
2 Tbsp. flour

1. Cook the dried beans until soft, or use canned beans for a quick start. If you are using a crock pot or slow cooker, you may have to add more water as the beans cook. When they are soft, drain the beans reserving 2 cups cooking water, and return the beans and reserved water to the pot. Add the rest of the ingredients, except the oil and flour, and simmer until tender.

2. In a sauté pan, bubble the oil and flour together over low heat until the flour starts to brown, then stir into the beans. Simmer until thickened and serve over rice.

Per cup: Calories: 177, Protein: 8 gm., Fat: 3 gm., Carbohydrates: 29 gm., Fiber 6 gm., Sodium: 496 mg.

FALAFEL

YIELD: ABOUT 24 ONE INCH BALLS

These falafels, made from cooked garbanzo beans rather than the bean flour, are easy to digest. They are baked in the oven rather than deep fried to reduce the fat content. Serve with chopped lettuce and tomato and a squirt of lemon on fat-free pita bread.

2 cloves fresh garlic
2 cups cooked garbanzo or fava beans, or 1-15 oz. can, drained
¼ cup water or bean cooking water
½ tsp. salt
¼ tsp. freshly ground black pepper
2 cups bread crumbs
½ cup onions, minced
¼ cup parsley, chopped
1 Tbsp. olive oil

1. Preheat the oven to 350°F.

2. With the food processor running, drop in and mince the garlic. Scrape the sides of the food processor down, add the garbanzo beans, water, salt, and black pepper, and process until creamy.

3. Stir the bean mixture into the bread crumbs, onions, and parsley.

4. Form into 1" balls. Spread the olive oil on a baking pan or spray with non-stick cooking spray. Bake for about 30 minutes, turning each ball carefully every 10 minutes until brown all sides.

Per ball: Calories: 61, Protein: 2 gm., Fat: 1 gm., Carbohydrates: 11 gm., Fiber 1 gm., Sodium: 107 mg.

LENTIL SPREAD OR PÂTÉ

YIELD: 4 CUPS

LENTIL SPREAD *can be served on crackers or bread as an appetizer or as an accompaniment to soup or salad.*

1 cup lentils
4 cups boiling water
¼ cup tomato paste
¼ tsp. allspice
1 medium onion, chopped
1 medium carrot, chopped
1 rib celery, chopped
2 cloves garlic, minced
½ tsp. thyme
2 Tbsp. soy sauce or tamari
⅛ tsp. red pepper flakes
1 cup toasted bread crumbs

1. Sort and wash the lentils, then add to the boiling water with the tomato paste and allspice. Simmer about 30 minutes.

2. Add the onion, carrot, celery, garlic, thyme, soy sauce, and red pepper flakes, and continue simmering until the vegetables are tender, the lentils are soft, and all the liquid has evaporated.

3. Cool and blend in a food processor with the toasted bread crumbs. Chill and serve.

Per 2 Tbsp.: Calories: 35, Protein: 2 gm., Fat: 0 gm., Carbohydrates: 6 gm., Fiber 1 gm., Sodium: 90 mg.

Bean Enchiladas

YIELD: ONE 11" X 7" PAN (4-6 SERVINGS)

Here is the always popular enchilada, saucy, vegan style. Add a green salad and SPANISH RICE (pg. 88) for a full meal. For a new taste treat, try using PINTO OR BLACK BEAN "REFRIES" (pg. 73) or NORTHERN ITALIAN "REFRIES" (pg. 71) for filling.

FOR *CHILI GRAVY:*
6 Tbsp. unbleached white
    flour
2 Tbsp. chili powder
1 Tbsp. onion powder
1 tsp. garlic powder
1 tsp. salt
½ tsp. cumin powder
3 cups water
¼ cup fresh cilantro,
    chopped

FOR *TOPPING:*
¼ cup water
1 large green pepper,
    chopped
1 large onion, chopped

FOR *FILLING:*
1½ cups pinto or black
    beans
6-5" corn or flour tortillas

1. Preheat the oven to 350°F.

2. Prepare the *CHILI GRAVY: Microwave Method:* In a large microwave-safe glass bowl or measuring cup, whip together the flour, chili powder, onion powder, garlic powder, salt, and cumin powder. Whip in the 3 cups water, microwave on high for about 6 minutes, then whip until smooth. Microwave again for 2 minutes or until it starts to boil and thicken slightly. Whip again until smooth. Whip in the cilantro and set aside. *Stovetop Method:* In a 2-quart saucepan, whip together the flour, chili powder, onion powder, garlic powder, salt, cumin powder, and water. Bring to a boil over medium heat, whipping to keep lumps from forming. Simmer and whip until thickened. Whip in the chopped fresh cilantro.

3. Prepare the *TOPPING: Microwave Method:* In another small microwave-safe container, microwave ¼ cup water, the green pepper, and onion on high for 4 minutes. *Stovetop Method:* Simmer the onion and green pepper in ¼ cup water over low heat until crisp tender.

4. Pour half the *CHILI GRAVY* into an 11" x 7" pan. Dip each tortilla into the remaining *CHILI GRAVY*, place it in the pan, fill with ¼ cup beans, and roll up the tortillas. Make a row across the pan. Pour the rest of the *CHILI GRAVY* over the top, sprinkle with the green peppers and onions, and bake for about 30 minutes or until hot.

Per serving: Calories: 198, Protein: 7 gm., Fat: 1 gm., Carbohydrates: 38 gm., Fiber 5 gm., Sodium: 430 mg.

NORTHERN ITALIAN "REFRIES"

YIELD: 3 CUPS

1 cup dried cannellini or
    Great Northern beans,
    or 1–16 oz. can
1 tsp. olive oil
1 medium onion, chopped
1 medium sweet yellow or
    green pepper, chopped
2 cloves garlic, minced
½ cup fresh parsley,
    chopped
½ tsp. sage
¼ tsp. rosemary
¼ tsp. thyme
⅛ tsp. freshly ground
    black pepper

1. Pressure cook the dried beans in 4 cups water for 60 minutes or until very soft, and drain.

2. Sauté all the other ingredients together until the onions are soft.

3. Blend all together until smooth. Serve hot with steamed vegetables or cold as a spread on crackers or bread.

Per 1/2 cup: Calories: 108, Protein: 6 gm., Fat: 1 gm., Carbohydrates: 19 gm., Fiber 4 gm., Sodium: 5 mg.

CAJUN STUFFED PEPPERS

YIELD: 6 SERVINGS

This is a good way to spice up leftover rice and beans. These peppers can be microwaved or baked in the oven. The list of ingredients may seem long, but this recipe is very quick to put together.

3 green, yellow, or red bell peppers
1 Tbsp. oil
2 Tbsp. unbleached white flour
½ tsp. salt
½ tsp. thyme
½ tsp. oregano
⅛ tsp. freshly ground black pepper
⅛ tsp. dry mustard
⅛ tsp. cayenne pepper
1 medium onion, chopped
1 small green pepper, chopped
1 stalk celery, chopped
2 cloves garlic, minced
¼ cup parsley, chopped
1-15 oz. can diced tomatoes
1 cup cooked red kidney beans
1 cup cooked rice

1. Cut the peppers in half, remove the seeds and membranes, and parboil for 10 minutes.

2. If you are going to bake in a conventional oven, preheat the oven to 350°F.

3. In a sauté pan, let the oil and flour bubble together over low heat until the flour starts to brown. Stir in the salt, thyme, oregano, black pepper, dry mustard, and cayenne pepper into the bubbling mixture. Stir in the onion, green pepper, celery, garlic, and parsley, and gently cook until tender. Mix in half the diced tomatoes and the beans and rice.

4. Stuff the pepper halves with the mixture, and arrange in a 2-quart glass baking dish surrounded with the rest of the diced tomatoes.

5. Microwave 5 to 10 minutes or bake in a conventional oven for 10 to 15 minutes until hot.

Per serving: Calories: 141, Protein: 5 gm., Fat: 2 gm., Carbohydrates: 24 gm., Fiber 5 gm., Sodium: 194 mg.

Pinto or Black Bean "Refries"

Yield: 4 cups

This takes about 5 minutes to whip together. For subtle changes in flavor and texture, try using cranberry, adzuki, anasazi, small red, or kidney beans as variations for the bean base of this dip. This recipe makes enough filling for a 9" x 13" pan of enchiladas.

3½ cups cooked pinto or
    black beans, or 2-16 oz.
    cans, drained
1-10 oz. can tomatoes and
    green chiles
½ cup fresh cilantro,
    chopped
2 cloves garlic, pressed
1 Tbsp. onion powder,
    or ¼ cup onion,
    chopped
1 tsp. salt

1. Blend all the ingredients together in a food processor or blender. Serve as burrito or enchilada filling, a dip or spread, or as a side dish.

Per 1/2 cup: Calories: 146, Protein: 7 gm., Fat: 0 gm., Carbohydrates: 28 gm., Fiber 6 gm., Sodium: 361 mg.

VARIATION: *BREAKFAST BURRITO:* For a hearty breakfast, spread ½ cup "refries" on a large fat-free flour tortilla, add salsa of choice to taste, roll up and enjoy.

CHILI BEANS

YIELD: 14 CUPS

If you're going to make a pot of CHILI BEANS, you might as well make a big one and freeze what you don't eat for later use. Freeze them in individual portions or in meal size portions for the family. This recipe gives the "open pot" method for cooking beans, which I think gives the best flavor. You can use any method you like for cooking the beans, or use canned or dehydrated instant beans for a really quick start. For this recipe you will need 8 cups of cooked beans.

4 cups dry pinto, kidney, red, or cranberry beans
water to cover (8–10 cups)
1-28 oz. can tomatoes (with juice), chopped
3 green peppers, chopped
2 onions, chopped
3 cloves garlic, minced
4 Tbsp. chili powder
2 tsp. salt
1 cup cilantro leaves, packed and chopped

1. Sort, rinse, and soak the beans overnight. Drain and rinse.

2. Gently boil the soaked beans, uncovered, until they are soft (about 2 to 3 hours). Keep the beans covered with liquid throughout the cooking time.

3. When the beans are soft, add the tomatoes, peppers, onions, garlic, chili powder, and salt. Simmer until the vegetables are tender, then stir in the cilantro leaves. Serve hot with bread, tortillas, or rice and a salad.

Per cup: Calories: 156, Protein: 8 gm., Fat: 0 gm., Carbohydrates: 30 gm., Fiber 6 gm., Sodium: 312 mg.

VARIATIONS: *CHILI BEANS WITH TEXTURED VEGETABLE PROTEIN:* With the vegetables, add 2 cups textured vegetable protein granules. Add more water to cover if needed.

Per cup: Calories: 193, Protein: 13 gm., Fat: 0 gm., Carbohydrates: 33 gm., Fiber 7 gm., Sodium: 315 mg.

CHILI BEANS WITH TOFU: Along with the vegetables, add 1 lb. tofu, which has been frozen, thawed, squeezed dry, and torn into bite sized pieces.

Per cup: Calories: 180, Protein: 10 gm., Fat: 1 gm., Carbohydrates: 31 gm., Fiber 6 gm., Sodium: 314 mg.

BLACK BEANS WITH TOMATO AND GREEN CHILES

YIELD: 3 CUPS

This makes a tasty, quick lunch or dinner served on fat-free pita bread with a green salad.

2 tsp. olive oil
½ cup onion, chopped
½ cup green pepper,
   chopped
1 clove garlic, minced
1-10 oz. can tomatoes and
   green chiles
2 cups cooked black beans,
     or 1-16 oz. can
¼ cup fresh cilantro,
   chopped

1. Sauté the onion, green pepper, and garlic in the olive oil until the onions are transparent. Stir in the tomatoes and green chiles, black beans, and cilantro. Heat thoroughly and serve in fat-free pita bread.

Per 1/2 cup: Calories: 103, Protein: 5 gm., Fat: 1 gm., Carbohydrates: 17 gm., Fiber 4 gm., Sodium: 5 mg.

VARIATION: Substitute garbanzo beans for black beans.

Per 1/2 cup: Calories: 117, Protein: 5 gm., Fat: 2 gm., Carbohydrates: 18 gm., Fiber 4 gm., Sodium: 9 mg.

SOY BURGERS

YIELD: 8 BURGERS

Use your leftover cooked soybeans to make these burgers or SOY NON-MEAT BALLS (see variation below). Serve SOY BURGERS on fat-free buns with mustard, lettuce, and tomato. SOY NON-MEAT BALLS are a great accompaniment to pasta.

2 cups cooked soybeans

½ cup uncooked rolled oats or whole wheat flour

½ cup oat bran or wheat germ

½ cup onion, finely chopped, or 2 tsp. onion powder

1 clove garlic, minced, or ½ tsp. garlic powder

2 Tbsp. tomato paste or ketchup

1 tsp. salt

½ tsp. oregano

½ tsp. basil

1. If you don't have leftover soy beans, pressure cook 1 cup unsoaked dried soybeans in 3 cups water for 60 to 75 minutes until they are so soft you can mash one on the roof of you mouth with your tongue. One cup dried beans yields about 2 cups cooked. Drain the soy beans and mash with a potato masher, or chop in the food processor.

2. Stir the mashed beans into the rest of the ingredients, mix well, and divide into 8 balls. Flatten each ball to about 1/2" thick or less. Fry on a non-stick surface sprayed with non-stick spray. Cook until browned on both sides.

Per burger: Calories: 130, Protein: 9 gm., Fat: 5 gm., Carbohydrates: 12 gm., Fiber 4 gm., Sodium: 270 mg.

VARIATION: *SOY NON-MEAT BALLS:* Form into 24 balls. Spray a 9" x 13" pan with non-stick spray or spread with 1 Tbsp. oil. Arrange the balls evenly in the pan, and bake at 350°F for 30 to 40 minutes, rolling the balls every 10 minutes to brown on all sides.

Per ball: Calories: 43, Protein: 3 gm., Fat: 1 gm., Carbohydrates: 4 gm., Fiber 1 gm., Sodium: 90 mg.

CHICK-PEA SPREAD

YIELD: 2 CUPS

Spread this savory spread on crackers or bread. It can be served as an appetizer or with soup or salad.

1 tsp. olive oil
1 medium onion, chopped
1 red bell pepper, chopped
2 cloves garlic, minced
2 cups cooked chick-peas,
    or 1-16 oz. can, drained
2 Tbsp. tomato paste
2 Tbsp. fresh parsley,
    chopped
½ tsp. salt
½ tsp. thyme
½ tsp. sage

1. Sauté the onion, red bell pepper, and garlic in the olive oil until soft.

2. Blend all the ingredients together in a food processor until smooth.

Per 2 Tbsp.: Calories: 43, Protein: 2 gm., Fat: 0 gm., Carbohydrates: 7 gm., Fiber 1 gm., Sodium: 70 mg.

MUJARADAH
(LENTILS AND RICE)

YIELD: 6 CUPS

This classic Middle Eastern combination of flavors makes a hearty breakfast, lunch or dinner.

1 Tbsp. olive oil
1 large onion, chopped
2 cloves garlic, minced
1 cup lentils
4 cups boiling water, vegetable bouillon or soup stock
1 cup long grain or basmati brown rice
¼ cup fresh parsley, or 1 Tbsp. dried
½ tsp. cumin
1 tsp. salt
¼ tsp. freshly ground black pepper

1. Sauté the onion and garlic in the olive oil.

2. Clean and rinse the lentils. When the onion is tender, stir in the lentils and boiling water. Bring to a boil, reduce the heat to a simmer, and cook for about 20 minutes.

3. Stir in the rice, parsley, cumin, salt, and black pepper. Cover and continue to simmer 40 minutes until both the rice and lentils are tender.

Per ½ cup: Calories: 123, Protein: 5 gm., Fat: 3 gm., Carbohydrates: 23 gm., Fiber 2 gm., Sodium: 181 mg.

MAINLY GRAINS

Whole grains are a mainstay of the vegan diet. Rich in protein, vitamins, minerals, and dietary fiber, whole grains are low in fat and of course, cholesterol free. There are a wide variety of familiar and new "gourmet" grains to choose from. Don't limit your menus to wheat, oats, corn, and rice. Choose from a broad range of flavors and textures including basmati brown rice, buckwheat, millet, quinoa (KEEN-wah), amaranth, wild rice, kamut, spelt, and a number of different specialty rices.

The dietary fiber in whole grains helps to lower the amount of fat and cholesterol that the body absorbs and helps to move food along through the digestive process. Fiber has been shown to help prevent gall stones and reduce the incidence of colon and rectal cancer by helping to absorb some cancer promoting substances.

Whole grains can be made savory or sweet and can be served at any meal in a variety of forms. The liquid added to cook the grains will change the flavor. Try using the cooking water left from vegetables, liquid drained from canned tomatoes or fruit, or the liquid from soaking dried mushrooms or fruit. Adding onions, garlic, and/or different combinations of herbs and spices will give a wide range of possible flavorings for grains. Grains can be served hot or cold, as a breakfast cereal, a salad, a hot side dish, a main course, in bread or other baked goods, in soup, or as a dessert.

Polenta with Roasted Red Bell Pepper Sauce

Yield: 3-4 servings (2½ cups sauce, four ½ cup servings polenta)

This brightly colored sauce freezes well if you want to make it ahead of time or make large batches while the peppers are plentiful. It is delicious with pasta as well.
The easiest, most foolproof way to cook polenta is in the microwave. This method is not traditional, but it eliminates all the watching over, stirring, and the dreaded lumping. The polenta can be made a day ahead and refrigerated. It can be molded in non-stick molds, cut out with cookie cutters for a more creative presentation, or simply cut into wedges from a cake or pie pan. The polenta and sauce can be reheated in the microwave just before serving. This recipe is featured on the cover.

FOR THE *POLENTA:*
2½ cups water
½ cup fine cornmeal or
   polenta
¼ tsp. salt (opt)

1. Prepare the *POLENTA:* Combine the water, cornmeal, and salt in a 2-quart glass bowl or measuring cup.

2. Microwave on high, uncovered, for 5 minutes. Remove and whip. Cover with plastic wrap, leaving a steam escape hole, and microwave again on high for 6 more minutes.

3. Whip again and pour into an 8" round pan, pie pan, or loaf pan to cool and become firm. If you have non-stick molds, pour in the hot polenta and cool until firm. The polenta should be about ½" thick.

FOR THE SAUCE:

2 lbs. red bell peppers
1 tsp. olive oil
1 large onion, chopped
3 garlic cloves, minced
½ cup water
¼ cup fresh basil
½ tsp. salt

1. Prepare the **ROASTED RED BELL PEPPER SAUCE:**: Preheat the oven to broil.

2. Wash the peppers and place under the broiler, turning until the skins are blackened all over. Place the blistered peppers in a plastic or heavy paper bag, close or seal the bag, and let stand for about 20 minutes. Peel off the skins, take out the membranes and seeds, and discard.

3. While the peppers are roasting, sauté the onion and garlic in the olive oil, adding water to keep from sticking if necessary. When the onions are transparent, add the basil and salt.

4. Process all the sauce ingredients together in a food processor or blender until smooth. Reheat the sauce and polenta in the microwave, and serve hot. Garnish with fresh basil leaves.

Per serving: Calories: 165, Protein: 4 gm., Fat: 2 gm., Carbohydrates: 32 gm., Fiber 6 gm., Sodium: 314 mg.

VARNISHKES

VARNISHKES are a savory treat featuring buckwheat or kasha. Buckwheat is not really wheat or even a true grain. It is the seed of a plant that is a relative of rhubarb.

1 tsp. olive oil
1 cup onion, chopped
1 cup buckwheat groats or
   kasha
2 cups boiling water
4 oz. pasta bow ties
1 tsp. salt

1. Sauté the onion in the olive oil for 2-3 minutes.

2. Stir in the buckwheat groats. Continue stirring until the mixture is dry looking (about 2 minutes), then pour in the boiling water. Reduce the heat to low, cover, and cook gently for 15 minutes.

3. While the buckwheat groats are cooking, cook the pasta bow ties in boiling water until tender.

4. Drain the pasta, fluff the buckwheat groats with a fork, and toss all together with salt to taste.

Per serving: Calories: 121, Protein: 3 gm., Fat: 1 gm., Carbohydrates: 23 gm., Fiber 2 gm., Sodium: 539 mg.

MINTED COUSCOUS
WITH GREEN ONIONS

YIELD: 4 CUPS

Couscous needs only boiling water and a few minutes to become a tender treat. It accommodates either savory or sweet flavoring.

1 tsp. oil
¼ tsp. turmeric
½ cup green onions,
   chopped
½ cup fresh or frozen green
   peas
1½ cups boiling water
½ tsp. salt
1 cup couscous
½ Tbsp. fresh mint, minced

1. Sauté the onions and turmeric in the oil. Add the peas, boiling water, and salt, return to a boil, and add the couscous. Cover, remove from the heat, and let stand 5-10 minutes.

2. Fluff and mix in the mint. Serve hot.

Per ½ cup: Calories: 60, Protein: 2 gm., Fat: 1 gm., Carbohydrates: 12 gm., Fiber 2 gm., Sodium: 136 mg.

BULGUR PILAF

YIELD: 3 CUPS

Serve this flavorful hearty whole grain pilaf for a side dish or a main dish.

2 tsp. olive oil
½ cup onions, chopped
1 clove garlic, minced
1 cup bulgur or cracked
 wheat
¼ tsp. basil
¼ tsp. oregano
2 cups boiling water
½ tsp. salt

1. Sauté the onions and garlic in the olive oil until the onions are transparent.

2. Stir in the bulgur or cracked wheat, basil, and oregano. Cook and stir until the grains start to brown slightly, then pour in the boiling water and salt. Cover, reduce heat to a simmer, and cook about 15 minutes or until the liquid is absorbed. Serve hot.

Per ½ cup: Calories: 113, Protein: 4 gm., Fat: 2 gm., Carbohydrates: 21 gm., Fiber 3 gm., Sodium: 180 mg.

VARIATION: Add 1 cup sliced mushrooms or chopped bell peppers to the sauté pan.

Per ½ cup: Calories: 116, Protein: 4 gm., Fat: 2 gm., Carbohydrates: 21 gm., Fiber 3 gm., Sodium: 181 mg.

SAFFRON RICE

YIELD: 3 CUPS

2 tsp. olive oil
1 clove garlic, crushed
1 small onion, chopped
   (about ½ cup)
1 cup brown or white
   basmati rice
2 cups boiling water
½ tsp. salt
1 pinch of saffron

1. Sauté the garlic and onion in the olive oil until the onion is transparent.

2. Add the uncooked rice to the pan, and stir fry for a few minutes to toast the rice.

3. Pour in the boiling water, salt, and saffron. Bring to a boil, turn the heat down to simmer, cover, and cook, undisturbed (45 minutes for brown rice or 20 minutes for white basmati rice).

Per ½ cup: Calories: 119, Protein: 2 gm., Fat: 2 gm., Carbohydrates: 23 gm., Fiber 1 gm., Sodium: 186 mg.

SAVORY MILLET

YIELD: ABOUT 3 CUPS

1 tsp. olive oil
1 sweet onion, chopped
1 clove garlic, minced
1 cup millet
1 tsp. summer savory
2 cups boiling water

1. Stir fry the onion, garlic, and millet in the olive oil briefly.

2. Add the savory and boiling water, cover, and steam over low heat 20 minutes until the water is absorbed. Serve hot.

Per ½ cup serving: Calories: 217, Protein: 6 gm., Fat: 3 gm., Carbohydrates: 41 gm., Fiber 6 gm., Sodium: 3 mg.

GLUTEN ROAST

Gluten is the protein part of wheat. It is the stretchy stuff that holds bread together.
GLUTEN ROAST *freezes well. Since it does require a long cooking time, I like to make 3 or*
4 pans at a time and freeze most of it for those times when I don't have time to cook. It is
delicious hot from the oven served with ROASTED ROOT VEGETABLES *(pg. 138). This is a*
basic recipe that can be incorporated into many different dishes. It can be sliced for hot
sandwiches, torn or cubed for stir fries, torn or chopped for burritos or enchiladas, or added
to soups or salads. One of my favorite ways is BARBECUE GLUTEN SANDWICHES *(pg. 87).*

1 Tbsp. soy sauce
1 Tbsp. olive oil
1 Tbsp. onion powder
1 tsp. garlic powder
¼ tsp. black pepper
enough water to make 1½
    cups liquid
1¾ cups vital wheat gluten
⅔ cup water
1 Tbsp. soy sauce
1 Tbsp. olive oil

1. Preheat the oven to 350°F.

2. Mix together 1 Tbsp. soy sauce, 1 Tbsp. olive oil, the onion powder, garlic powder, black pepper, and enough water to make 1½ cups liquid.

3. Stir the liquid into the vital wheat gluten until it is well mixed, and the liquid is absorbed.

4. In another bowl, mix together ⅔ cup water, 1 Tbsp. soy sauce, and 1 Tbsp. olive oil. Pour half the liquid into a loaf pan. Stretch, pull, and push the gluten to fit into the pan. Pour the rest of the liquid over the gluten, cover, and bake for about 75 minutes.

Per serving: Calories: 174, Protein: 29 gm., Fat: 5 gm., Carbohydrates: 5 gm., Fiber 0 gm., Sodium: 287 mg.

Gluten Barbecue Sandwiches

YIELD: 4 SANDWICHES

Serve this Barbecue hot or cold, either in a sandwich or as an entrée. This is a sandwich with a chewy texture and a spicy sauce.

½ loaf GLUTEN ROAST
(pg. 86)
1 cup of your favorite non-
fat barbecue sauce

1. Slice the **GLUTEN ROAST** very thin in a food processor or slicer.

2. Mix the sliced gluten together with the barbecue sauce, and heat in the microwave or on the stovetop.

3. Serve on toasted buns or between slices of low-fat or fat-free bread.

Per serving (barbecue only): Calories: 328, Protein: 26 gm., Fat: 3 gm., Carbohydrates: 40 gm., Fiber 0 gm., Sodium: 268 mg.

Per sandwich (with 2 slices low-fat whole wheat bread): Calories: 450, Protein: 30 gm., Fat: 3 gm., Carbohydrates: 75 gm., Fiber 3 gm., Sodium: 270 mg.

SPANISH RICE

This is a quick and easy dish, especially if you have left over rice in the refrigerator.

1 tsp. olive oil
1 Tbsp. water
1 small onion, chopped
½ green pepper, chopped
1 clove garlic, crushed
3 cups cooked brown rice
1 cup tomato sauce or
    crushed tomatoes
2 tsp. chili powder
1 tsp. salt
½ cup cilantro, chopped

1. *Stovetop Method:* Sauté the onion, green pepper, and garlic in the olive oil and water in a sauté pan until the onions are transparent. *Microwave Method:* Microwave the onion, green pepper, and garlic in the olive oil and water on high, covered, for about 3 minutes.

2. Mix in the cooked rice, tomato sauce, chili powder, salt, and cilantro.

3. Continue heating on the stovetop, or microwave again on high until heated through. Serve hot.

Per serving: Calories: 146, Protein: 3 gm., Fat: 1 gm., Carbohydrates: 30 gm., Fiber 3 gm., Sodium: 373 mg.

CHILEQUILES

YIELD: 3 CUPS (4-6 SERVINGS)

Chilequiles can be served at any meal. They can be made anywhere from mild to fiery hot depending on the type of salsa you use. Use the microwave for a soft texture and the oven for crispy.

¾ cup salsa of choice (non-fat)
½ lb. reduced-fat tofu, crumbled
6-12 corn tortillas, cut in sixths
½ tsp. salt

1. *Microwave Method:* Toss the salsa, tofu, tortillas, and salt together in a microwave-safe bowl. Cover and microwave on high for 3 minutes until hot. Serve hot.

2. *Oven Method:* Preheat the oven to 400°F. Spread the tortilla pieces on a baking sheet, and bake until crispy and light brown. Mix together the salsa, tofu, and salt. Toss together with the tortilla pieces and spread on the cookie sheet again. Bake for about 5 more minutes or until heated through. Serve hot.

Per serving: Calories: 174, Protein: 9 gm., Fat: 4 gm., Carbohydrates: 26 gm., Fiber 4 gm., Sodium: 578 mg.

GRAIN BURGERS

YIELD: NINE 3" BURGERS

This is a tasty, quick way to enjoy the use of leftover cooked grains.

½ cup wheat germ
½ cup plum tomatoes,
    peeled and chopped
2 cups cooked brown rice
    or other leftover cooked
    grain
1 cup uncooked rolled oats
½ tsp. garlic
1 small onion
1-2 Tbsp. nutritional yeast
½ tsp. salt
1 Tbsp. oil

1. Mix together all the ingredients except the oil.

2. Form into 9 burgers and brown on a non-stick griddle with non-stick spray, or grill using 1 Tbsp. oil.

3. Serve on fat-free buns with all the fixings.

Per burger: Calories: 131, Protein: 5 gm., Fat: 4 gm., Carbohydrates: 21 gm., Fiber 3 gm., Sodium: 121 mg.

TAMALE DUMPLINGS

YIELD: 20-24 DUMPLINGS (6-8 SERVINGS)

Try steaming these dumplings in the broth of pinto or black beans or CHILI BEANS (pg. 74). Make sure there is plenty of liquid. You can replace the cornmeal and flour with masa harina.

½ cup cornmeal
½ cup unbleached white
　flour
2 tsp. baking powder
½ tsp. salt
½ cup water
2 tsp. oil
1 small jalapeño, chopped
　(opt)

1. Mix the dry ingredients together. Mix the water and oil, stir in the jalapeños, and pour into the dry ingredients. Stir just until the dry ingredients are moistened.

2. Drop by spoonfuls into simmering liquid (soup or stock), and steam, covered, without lifting the lid to peek, for about 15 minutes. Serve immediately.

Per serving: Calories: 76, Protein: 2 gm., Fat: 1 gm., Carbohydrates: 14 gm., Fiber 1 gm., Sodium: 152 mg.

MOROCCAN VEGETABLES
WITH COUSCOUS

YIELD: 6 SERVINGS

This is a quick and exotic, one-pot meal. Have all the vegetables cut and ready to go before starting to cook.

2 tsp. olive oil
2 cloves garlic, minced
1 small onion
¼ lb. carrots, cut in ¼"
　　slices
¼ lb. turnips, cut in ½"
　　chunks
¼ lb. zucchini, cut in ½"
　　chunks
¼ lb. yellow summer
　　squash, cut in ½" chunks
¼ lb. savory cabbage, cut in
　　1" chunks
3 oz. prunes, cut in halves
　　(½ cup)
1 tsp. gingerroot, minced
1 tsp. salt
½ tsp. crushed red pepper
½ tsp. cinnamon
¼ tsp. cumin
¼ tsp. turmeric
2 cups boiling water
1 cup couscous

1. Sauté the garlic and onion in the olive oil until transparent. Add the carrots and turnips, stir, cover, and simmer over low heat for about 8 minutes.

2. Add the rest of the vegetables and spices, stir, cover, and simmer about 5 more minutes or until all the vegetables are tender. Turn off the heat.

3. Pour in the boiling water, move the vegetables aside, and pour in the couscous so that it is covered by the water. Cover the pot and let set for about 5 minutes or until the couscous has absorbed all the water. Fluff the couscous and serve hot.

Per serving: Calories: 143, Protein: 3 gm., Fat: 1 gm., Carbohydrates: 29 gm., Fiber 5 gm., Sodium: 386 mg.

FOCACCIA

YIELD: 8 SLICES

Although this takes some time to prepare, the result is well worth it.

1 Tbsp. active dry yeast
1 cup warm water
1 Tbsp. sweetener of choice
1 Tbsp. olive oil
½ tsp. salt
2 cups whole wheat pastry flour
1 cup unbleached white flour
½ cup plum tomatoes, seeded and chopped
1 Tbsp. fresh basil, finely chopped
¼ cup onions, finely chopped
1 clove garlic, finely minced
½ green pepper, finely chopped

1. Sprinkle the yeast over the warm water, and let it soften and dissolve for about 5 minutes.

2. Beat in the sweetener, olive oil, and salt with a heavy duty mixer or wooden spoon. Add the whole wheat pastry flour, and beat until dough is smooth and elastic. Add the unbleached flour, and beat and knead until smooth and elastic. Cover the dough in a lightly oiled bowl, and let it rise in a warm place until double in bulk.

3. Preheat the oven to 450°F.

4. Punch down the dough and knead briefly. Lightly oil a 12" round pizza pan. Roll and stretch the dough to fit the pan. Punch holes in the dough about every inch over the pan with the end of a wooden spoon or chop stick.

5. Sprinkle the tomatoes, basil, onions, garlic, and green pepper over the top. Let rise again about 15 minutes, then bake for about 12 minutes or until browned. Cut into wedges and serve.

Per slice: Calories: 182, Protein: 6 gm., Fat: 2 gm., Carbohydrates: 34 gm., Fiber 4 gm., Sodium: 138 mg.

EGGLESS WHOLE GRAIN PANCAKES

YIELD: 12 PANCAKES

1½ cups whole wheat flour
½ cup cornmeal
1 Tbsp. baking powder
2 cups fat-free soymilk

1. Preheat a non-stick griddle.

2. In a mixing bowl, mix together the flour, cornmeal, and baking powder. Stir in the soymilk just until everything is moistened. Spray the griddle with non-stick spray and pour on the pancakes. When they bubble up, flip them over and bake until browned. Serve with jelly or syrup.

Per pancake: Calories: 88, Protein: 4 gm., Fat: 0 gm., Carbohydrates: 18 gm., Fiber 2 gm., Sodium: 97 mg.

EGGLESS APPLESAUCE-BRAN MUFFINS

YIELD: 12 MUFFINS

2 cups whole wheat flour
1½ cup oat bran
1½ tsp. baking soda
2 cups unsweetened apple sauce
½ cup sorghum syrup or honey
½ cup raisins

1. Preheat oven to 400°F.

2. In a mixing bowl, mix together the flour, bran, baking soda and raisins. Make a well in the middle of the dry ingredients and pour in the apple sauce and sorghum. Mix together just until everything is moistened. Spray a non-stick muffin pan with non-stick spray and pour the batter into 12 muffins. Bake for 20 to 25 minutes.

Per muffin: Calories: 126, Protein: 4 gm., Fat: 1 gm., Carbohydrates: 31 gm., Fiber 3 gm., Sodium: 160 mg.

MAINLY PASTA

Pasta comes in so many different shapes and forms, there is truly something for everyone. Unaccompanied, most pastas are a low-fat food (about 1 to 2 grams per 2 oz. serving) and a good source of protein, fiber, and complex carbohydrates. Whole grain pastas provide more protein, vitamins, minerals, and fiber than those made with processed grains. They are all quick to prepare and easy to digest. There are a wide variety of sauces and accompaniments for versatile and tasty meals.

Some more exotic pastas combine wheat with Jerusalem artichoke flour, quinoa (KEEN-wah), sesame, soy flour, vegetables, or herbs for unique flavors and textures. If you have wheat allergies, try pasta made from corn flour, buckwheat flour, spelt flour, or rice flour.

Pasta's reputation as a high-fat food comes from the caloric-rich sauces that traditionally are served with it. With a luscious light sauce, pasta can be a quick, tasty, and satisfying low-fat treat for a snack or a meal.

Rigatoni Poblano

YIELD: 4 SERVINGS

This delicious, colorful pasta freezes well.

2 poblano peppers
8 oz. rigatoni
1 tsp. olive oil
1 large onion, chopped
2 cloves garlic, minced or pressed
2 cups tomatoes, peeled, seeded, and chopped, or 1-16 oz. can diced tomatoes
2 Tbsp. fresh basil, chopped, or 2 tsp. dried basil
grated non-fat soy Parmesan cheese substitute, (opt) or nutritional yeast (opt)

1. Roast the poblanos over a flame or under the broiler until charred and blistered all over. Close the peppers in a paper or plastic bag for 15 to 20 minutes, then peel, remove the membranes and seeds, and chop.

2. Cook the rigatoni according to the package directions. Rinse, drain, and keep hot.

3. While the pasta is cooking, sauté the onion and garlic in the olive oil. When the onions are transparent, stir in the tomatoes, basil, and roasted peppers. Cook only briefly to heat, then toss with the hot pasta. Sprinkle the top of each serving with the grated Parmesan cheese substitute or nutritional yeast, and serve.

Per serving: Calories: 116, Protein: 4 gm., Fat: 1 gm., Carbohydrates: 22 gm., Fiber 4 gm., Sodium: 12 mg.

Pasta Frittata

YIELD: 6-8 SERVINGS

Serve this frittata with CHUNKY MARINARA *(pg. 99) and a* MIXED GREEN SALAD *(pg. 42) for a full meal. This is a colorful and flavorful way to use up left over pasta.*

½ lb. angel hair pasta or spaghetti
2 tsp. olive oil
1 medium onion (½ lb.), chopped
3 cloves garlic, minced
¼ lb. green peppers, chopped
2 oz. fresh basil, chopped
2 oz. fresh Italian parsley, chopped
½ lb. reduced-fat tofu
1 tsp. salt
¼ tsp. freshly ground black pepper
½ cup black olives, chopped (opt)
2 Tbsp. capers chopped (opt)

1. Cook the pasta according to the package directions, rinse, and drain.

2. Preheat the oven to 350°F.

3. Sauté the onion, garlic, and green peppers in 1 tsp. olive oil over low heat until the onion is transparent, then mix in the basil and parsley.

4. In a food processor or blender, blend the tofu, salt, and black pepper until smooth and creamy. Fold in the olives and capers.

5. Oil a 9" pie pan with 1 tsp. olive oil. Mix all the ingredients together, press into the oiled pie pan, and bake for 30 minutes. Let cool for a few minutes before cutting into wedges.

Per serving: Calories: 111, Protein: 6 gm., Fat: 3 gm., Carbohydrates: 15 gm., Fiber 2 gm., Sodium: 312 mg.

Basic Marinara Sauce

YIELD: ABOUT 4½ CUPS

This fat-free basic Italian tomato sauce can be served as is for a chunky sauce or blended when cooled for a smooth sauce. This is enough sauce for ½ lb. pasta.

½ cup water
1 medium onion, chopped
1 small green pepper, chopped
2 cloves garlic, crushed
1 small carrot, chopped
¼ cup fresh parsley, chopped
1-28 oz. can crushed tomatoes
½ cup fresh basil leaves, chopped, or 1 tsp. dried basil
2 Tbsp. fresh oregano leaves, chopped, or ¼ tsp. dried oregano
1 tsp. salt
¼ tsp. freshly ground black pepper

1. Simmer the onion, green pepper, garlic, carrot, and parsley together in the water until almost tender.

2. Add the tomatoes, basil, oregano, salt, and black pepper, and simmer for about 20 minutes. Cool and blend until smooth in a food processor or blender.

Per ½ cup: Calories: 30, Protein: 1 gm., Fat: 0 gm., Carbohydrates: 6 gm., Fiber 2 gm., Sodium: 281 mg.

VARIATIONS: *MUSHROOM MARINARA:* Add 1 lb. sliced mushrooms of choice to the simmering sauce.

Per ½ cup: Calories: 44, Protein: 2 gm., Fat: 0 gm., Carbohydrates: 9 gm., Fiber 3 gm., Sodium: 282 mg.

MARINARA WITH TEXTURED VEGETABLE PROTEIN: Add 1 cup granular or flake textured vegetable protein to the simmering sauce.

Per ½ cup: Calories: 62, Protein: 6 gm., Fat: 0 gm., Carbohydrates: 9 gm., Fiber 3 gm., Sodium: 283 mg.

CHUNKY FRESH MARINARA

YIELD: 3 CUPS

For a quick and easy meal, serve this colorful, chunky sauce over spinach fettuccini along with a fresh green salad and a crusty bread. The sauce is especially flavorful made with fresh produce at the height of the season but also works well with canned tomatoes any time of the year. This sauce freezes well.

6 oz. spinach fettuccini
1 Tbsp. olive oil
1 large onion, chopped
1 large yellow or green
  bell pepper, chopped
3 cloves fresh garlic, minced
2 cups tomatoes, diced and
  seeded, or 1-16 oz. can
  diced tomatoes
½ cup fresh basil, packed
  and then chopped
½ tsp. salt

1. Cook the fettuccini until tender according to the package directions.

2. Sauté the onion, bell pepper, and garlic in the olive oil over low heat until the onion is transparent.

3. Stir in the tomatoes, basil, and salt, and simmer until hot. The longer you simmer, the more the flavors meld. Serve over hot pasta.

Per ½ cup sauce: Calories: 49, Protein: 1 gm., Fat: 2 gm., Carbohydrates: 6 gm., Fiber 2 gm., Sodium: 185 mg.

Per ½ cup sauce with 1 oz. fettuccini: Calories: 84, Protein: 2 gm., Fat: 2 gm., Carbohydrates: 13 gm., Fiber 2 gm., Sodium: 188 mg.

ORZO SHIITAKE PILAF

YIELD: 5 CUPS

If you can't find fresh shiitake mushrooms, you can substitute another type of fresh mushroom or soak dried shiitake mushrooms, using the soaking water as part or all of the cooking water.

2 tsp. olive oil
½ lb. onions, chopped
¼ lb. sweet red bell pepper, chopped
¼ lb. fresh shiitake, sliced
2½ cups boiling water
½ lb. orzo (about 1¼ cups)
1 tsp. salt
⅛ tsp. freshly ground black pepper
¼ cup fresh parsley, chopped

1. Sauté the onions, bell pepper, and shiitake in the olive oil until the onions are transparent.

2. Add the rest of the ingredients, cover, and simmer about 15 minutes until the water is absorbed. Fluff and serve.

Per ½ cup: Calories: 51, Protein: 2 gm., Fat: 1 gm., Carbohydrates: 9 gm., Fiber 2 gm., Sodium: 216 mg.

FUSILLI E FAGIOLI

YIELD: 8 CUPS

Add a salad for a quick and easy meal.

1 Tbsp. olive oil
1 cup onion, chopped
1 cup green pepper,
    chopped
2 cloves garlic
¼ oz. fresh basil, chopped
1 Tbsp. fresh oregano, or
    1 tsp. dry oregano
2-16 oz. cans diced
    tomatoes
1-16 oz. can navy or white
    kidney beans
1 tsp. salt
¼ tsp. freshly ground black
    pepper
8 oz. fusilli, cooked and
drained

1. Sauté the onion, green pepper, garlic, basil, and oregano in the olive oil.

2. Toss together with the rest of the ingredients, heat through, and serve.

Per ½ cup: Calories: 78, Protein: 3 gm., Fat: 1 gm., Carbohydrates: 14 gm., Fiber 3 gm., Sodium: 139 mg.

Lasagne with Two Fillings

Yield: one 9" x 13" pan (8-12 servings)

FOR *TOFU FILLING:*
¾ lb. reduced-fat tofu
½ Tbsp. onion powder
½ tsp. salt
½ tsp. basil
¼ tsp. garlic powder

FOR *TEXTURED VEGETABLE
PROTEIN FILLING:*
⅞ cup boiling water
1 cup textured vegetable
    protein granules
1 tsp. olive oil
1 onion, chopped
1 green pepper, chopped
2 cloves garlic, minced
1 tsp. basil
½ tsp. oregano
1 Tbsp. soy sauce

4 cups BASIC MARINARA
    SAUCE (pg. 98)
12 lasagne noodles (½ lb.)
4 oz. non-fat soy
    mozzarella cheese sub-
    stitute, grated (opt)

1. Prepare the *TOFU FILLING:* Blend all the ingredients in a food processor or blender until smooth.

2. Prepare the *TEXTURED VEGETABLE PROTEIN FILLING:* Pour the boiling water over the textured vegetable protein, and let stand for about 10 minutes. While the textured vegetable protein is standing, sauté the onion, green pepper, garlic, basil, and oregano in the olive oil. Add the hydrated textured vegetable protein and soy sauce, and stir fry for a few minutes.

3. Assemble the LASAGNE: Cook the lasagne noodles according to the directions on the package, and drain. Spread 1 cup MARINARA SAUCE over the bottom of a 9" x 13" pan. Cover the sauce with 4 cooked lasagne noodles, and spread the *TOFU FILLING* evenly over the noodles. Cover with 4 more cooked lasagne noodles and about 1½ cups sauce, then spread the *TEXTURED VEGETABLE PROTEIN FILLING* evenly over the layer of sauce. Cover with 4 more cooked lasagne noodles, and the rest of the sauce, then cover evenly with the grated non-fat soy mozzarella cheese substitute.

4. Bake covered for about 30 minutes, then uncover for the last 5 minutes of baking.

Per serving: Calories: 223, Protein: 14 gm., Fat: 3 gm., Carbohydrates: 36 gm., Fiber 4 gm., Sodium: 225 mg.

MEXICAN MACARONI

YIELD: 6 CUPS

This is a quick and easy fusion of flavors.

2 cups water
2 Tbsp. tomato paste
1 Tbsp. chili powder
2 tsp. onion powder
½ tsp. garlic powder
1 tsp. salt
1 cup textured vegetable
   protein, or 1 lb. frozen
   tofu, thawed, squeezed
   dry, and torn into bite
   size pieces
½ lb. macaroni (elbows or
   shells)

1. Mix the water, tomato paste, chili powder, onion powder, garlic powder, and salt together in a saucepan. Stir in the textured vegetable protein or frozen tofu, and simmer for 20 minutes.

2. Cook the macaroni according to the package directions, rinse, and drain. Mix all together and serve hot.

Per cup: Calories: 90, Protein: 8 gm., Fat: 0 gm., Carbohydrates: 13 gm., Fiber 2 gm., Sodium: 363 mg.

SPRING FRITTATA

This frittata combines a creamy spring green color with a delightful savory taste.

1-10 oz. pkg. frozen
  spinach
2 oz. flat noodles
1 tsp. olive oil
¼ cup water
1 large sweet onion (about
  1½ cups), chopped
2 cloves garlic, minced
½ lb. reduced-fat tofu
1 Tbsp. sweet miso
¼ tsp. freshly ground black
  pepper
¼ tsp. freshly ground
  nutmeg

1. Thaw and drain the spinach in a colander for 30 minutes

2. Preheat the oven to 350°F.

3. Boil the noodles until tender but firm. Rinse, drain, and set aside.

4. Sauté the onion and garlic in the olive oil and water.

5. Blend the tofu, miso, black pepper, and nutmeg in a food processor or blender until creamy. Fold in the spinach, noodles, and the onion and garlic together and pour into a non-stick pie or tart pan. Bake for about 30 minutes or until set. Invert on to a serving plate to serve.

Per serving: Calories: 85, Protein: 5 gm., Fat: 2 gm., Carbohydrates: 11 gm., Fiber 3 gm., Sodium: 52 mg.

ROASTED PEPPER WITH SOMEN

Somen is an oriental pasta similar to angel hair.

1 sweet yellow bell pepper
1 sweet red bell pepper
1 poblano pepper
6 oz. somen
1 cup vegetable stock
2 Tbsp. soy sauce
1 Tbsp. cornstarch or
   arrowroot
1 Tbsp. sweetener of choice
1 tsp. toasted sesame oil
2 cloves garlic, minced

1. Roast the peppers under the broiler or over a flame until charred evenly. Close the charred peppers in a paper or plastic bag for 15 to 20 minutes. Remove the skins, seeds, and membranes from the peppers, and discard. Cut the peppers into long strips.

2. Cook the somen according to package directions until tender. Rinse, drain, and keep hot.

3. *Stovetop Method:* In a saucepan, mix together the vegetable stock, soy sauce, cornstarch, sweetener, sesame oil, and garlic, then simmer and stir over low heat until thickened. *Microwave Method:* Whip together the vegetable stock, soy sauce, cornstarch, sweetener, sesame oil, and garlic in a microwave-safe bowl. Microwave on high for 2 minutes, or until thickened, and whip again.

4. Toss all together and serve.

Per serving: Calories: 93, Protein: 3 gm., Fat: 1 gm., Carbohydrates: 18 gm., Fiber 1 gm., Sodium: 404 mg.

TOFU-SPINACH LASAGNE FLOWERS

YIELD: 24 FLOWERS (8-12 SERVINGS)

Try this for a delicious and unique presentation of lasagne. This large recipe freezes well.

12 lasagne noodles (about 12 oz.)

FOR FILLING:
½ cup water
1 large sweet onion, chopped
3 cloves garlic, minced
2 bunches fresh spinach, washed, stemmed, and chopped, or 2-10 oz. pkgs. frozen chopped spinach, thawed and drained
2 lbs. firm reduced-fat tofu
1 Tbsp. onion powder
½ tsp. garlic powder
1 tsp. salt
¼ tsp. freshly ground black pepper

2 cups BASIC MARINARA SAUCE (pg. 98), or 1-15 oz. can or jar fat-free tomato sauce

1. Preheat the oven to 350°F.

2. Cook the lasagne noodles according to the package directions, rinse, and drain.

3. Prepare the *FILLING*: Sauté the onion and garlic in the water until soft. If using fresh spinach, gently steam over low heat until wilted. If using frozen spinach, thaw and drain. When the onion is tender, stir in the spinach, cover, and turn off the heat. Blend the tofu, onion powder, garlic powder, salt, and black pepper in a food processor until it is the consistency of ricotta cheese. Fold the tofu and spinach mixtures together.

4. Lay the cooked lasagne noodles out flat on a board or counter, and spread about ½ cup of the filling along the length of each noodle. Roll up each noodle and cut crosswise into halves that look like flowers when stood up on the cut end.

5. Pour the BASIC MARINARA SAUCE into a 9" x 13" pan, and arrange the lasagne flowers in rows of 4, cut-side down, in the sauce. Cover and bake for about 30 minutes until hot and bubbly.

Per serving: Calories: 257, Protein: 17 gm., Fat: 5 gm., Carbohydrates: 37 gm., Fiber 7 gm., Sodium: 566 mg.

MAINLY TOFU, TEMPEH, AND TEXTURED VEGETABLE PROTEIN

Tofu, tempeh, and textured vegetable protein are vegetarian fast foods. These versatile foods are made from soybeans and contain high-quality, complete protein. (Tempeh can also be made from grains or a mixture of grains, beans, and/or nuts.) All of these soy products are processed by different methods, making them easier to digest and quicker to cook.

Tofu is the cheese made from soymilk. High in protein, calcium, iron, vitamin E, and B vitamins, tofu is very low in saturated fat. The fat found in tofu is mostly "good" fat (monounsaturated), and there are reduced-fat and "lite" varieties of tofu available on the market. Up until recently, the soybean has been mainly used for oil in the west, but a low-fat soybean is in the works. The recipes in this book call for either "reduced-fat" tofu or "lite" silken tofu. Reduced-fat tofu is made by traditional methods and can be found in the refrigerated section of your market. It should be stored in the refrigerator under cold water, which should be changed every day until the tofu is used. Tofu will keep about a week under these conditions. Lite silken tofu can be found on the shelf in aseptic packaging, and needs no refrigeration until opened. Once it is opened, the unused portion should be treated the same as traditional tofu.

Tempeh is a cultured food usually made from soybeans. The culture breaks down the trypsin inhibitors in the bean and helps make it digestible. It has a nutty, savory flavor and is usually stored in the freezer.

For the recipes in this book, tempeh must be steamed for 20 minutes before it is ready to eat. It can be grilled, fried, or simmered further for varied flavor and texture.

Textured vegetable protein is an extruded, dehydrated soy food made from soybeans after the oil has been extracted. It is very low in fat and calories and high in protein, fiber, and potassium. It is available in several sizes, including small granules or flakes, chunks, and even steaks. Since it is already precooked, it is a very quick and easy protein source to work with.

Don't shy away from tofu or tempeh because of the high percentage of calories from fat in the soybean. These foods are rarely eaten alone, and their companion ingredients bring the overall calories from fat in a dish way down. The wealth of flavor and variety they bring to the vegetarian diet is well worth any fat calorie balancing that may need to be done. Remember, it is not any one day or meal that makes the difference, it is an over all balanced diet that promotes good health.

More tofu, tempeh, and textured vegetable protein recipes can be found in SNACKS AND APPETIZERS, PASTA, SALADS AND DRESSINGS, and LIGHTER SWEET THINGS sections.

FAJITAS WITH TEXTURED VEGETABLE PROTEIN

YIELD: 6 FAJITAS

These sizzling, colorful, and tasty fajitas are featured on the cover. They are a quick and easy meal for anytime.

1 Tbsp. wine vinegar
1 Tbsp. soy sauce
½ tsp. garlic powder, or
    1 clove garlic, minced
¾ cup boiling water
1 cup chunk style textured
    vegetable protein
1 onion, cut in rings
3 bell peppers, cut in slices
    (for more color use red,
    yellow, and green bell
    peppers)
6 flour or corn tortillas

1. Mix together the wine vinegar, soy sauce, and garlic powder. Add the boiling water and pour over the textured vegetable protein. Cover and let stand for about 15 minutes.

2. Grill the soaked textured vegetable protein on a hot, non-stick griddle along with the onion rings and bell pepper slices. Use a non-stick spray on the grill as needed. Sprinkle with the remaining soaking liquid while cooking.

3. Warm each flour or corn tortillas on the hot griddle for only a few seconds until soft.

4. Serve hot with SALSA FRESCA (pg. 21) or your favorite salsa. Let the individual put each fajita together to taste.

Per fajita: Calories: 129, Protein: 9 gm., Fat: 1 gm., Carbohydrates: 20 gm., Fiber 3 gm., Sodium: 174 mg.

CHIPOTLE CORN CUSTARD

YIELD: ONE 9" PIE (6-8 SERVINGS)

Smoky flavored chipotle chile and fresh cilantro give this colorful dish its unique flavor. This could be a main dish or a side dish, depending on what you serve it with. It is very quick to whip together.

1 tsp. olive oil (opt)
1 Tbsp. water
2 cloves garlic, crushed
1 medium onion, chopped
1 red bell pepper, chopped
1 green bell pepper, chopped
2 cups fresh or frozen corn, or 1-16 oz. can, drained
¼ cup fresh cilantro, chopped
2-10.5 oz. pkgs. lite silken tofu
1 tsp. salt
½ tsp. crushed chipotle

1. Preheat the oven to 350°F.

2. *Microwave Method:* In a microwave-safe bowl, mix together the olive oil, water, garlic, onion, bell peppers, corn, and cilantro. Cover and microwave on high for about 4 minutes. Stir again, cover, and microwave 4 more minutes. *Stovetop Method:* Sauté the garlic, onion, bell peppers, corn, and cilantro in the olive oil and water until tender.

3. While the vegetables are cooking, blend together the tofu, salt, and chipotle in a food processor or blender until smooth and creamy.

4. Mix all the ingredients together, and pour into a 9" pie or quiche pan. Bake for about 1 hour or until set.

Per cup: Calories: 88, Protein: 7 gm., Fat: 1 gm., Carbohydrates: 13 gm., Fiber 3 gm., Sodium: 389 mg.

HEARTY TEMPEH STEW

YIELD: 7-8 CUPS

A savory, warm comfort food for a cold winters day.

8 oz. tempeh
2 Tbsp. soy sauce
2 cloves garlic, minced
4 cups water
1 bay leaf
½ lb. carrots, cut in ¾"
   chunks
½ lb. potatoes, cut in ¾"
   chunks
¼ lb. onions, cut in ¾"
   chunks
1 Tbsp. olive oil
⅓ cup unbleached white
   flour or whole wheat
   pastry flour
½ tsp. thyme
½ tsp. sage
¼ cup fresh parsley,
   chopped
½ lb. fresh snow peas,
   stemmed, or frozen,
   thawed

1. Steam the tempeh for 20 minutes. While the tempeh is steaming, mix together the soy sauce and garlic, then prepare the vegetables. Cut the steamed tempeh into 3/4" chunks, lay in a flat pan and pour the soy sauce and garlic mixture over.

2. In a saucepan, heat the water to boiling, add the bay leaf, carrots, potatoes, and onions, and simmer until tender (about 10 minutes).

3. While the vegetables are cooking, brown the tempeh in the olive oil in a non-stick pan. When the tempeh is browned, remove it from the pan, add the flour, and lightly brown. Whip about 2 cups of the vegetable cooking water into the browned flour until smooth and thickened into a gravy. Stir the gravy into the vegetables, leaving no lumps. Add the browned tempeh, thyme, sage, parsley, and snow peas, and simmer until the snow peas are just tender. Serve hot.

Per serving: Calories: 166, Protein: 8 gm., Fat: 5 gm., Carbohydrates: 24 gm., Fiber 5 gm., Sodium: 314 mg.

BROILED TOFU OR TEMPEH

This is a basic recipe that can be varied by adding other herbs or spices to taste. Serve the BROILED TOFU OR TEMPEH *accompanied with any salsa (see* SNACKS & APPETIZERS *section) or sauce of your choice, as a main dish, or in a sandwich.*

1 lb. reduced-fat tofu or
   tempeh
2 Tbsp. soy sauce
2 Tbsp. water
1 tsp. fresh ginger, grated
½ tsp. garlic powder
⅛ tsp. red pepper flakes
   (opt)
nutritional yeast (opt)
non-stick olive oil baking
   spray

1. Steam the tempeh for 20 minutes. Cut the tofu or tempeh in to 3/8" thick slices, pat dry, and lay out in a glass pan.

2. Mix together the rest of the ingredients, except the nutritional yeast, and pour over the slices.

3. Spray a shallow baking pan with non-stick spray, and lay out the flavored slices. Broil until browned (about 3 minutes), turn, sprinkle with nutritional yeast, and broil until browned on the second side (about 2 more minutes).

Tofu per serving: Calories: 119, Protein: 13 gm., Fat: 5 gm., Carbohydrates: 6 gm., Fiber 3 gm., Sodium: 509 mg.

Tempeh per serving: Calories: 88, Protein: 8 gm., Fat: 3 gm., Carbohydrates: 8 gm., Fiber 2 gm., Sodium: 505 mg.

GINGER BRAISED TOFU

For the fullest flavor, marinate the tofu overnight. If you are in a rush, it is still flavorful with the marinating time eliminated.

1 lb. reduced-fat tofu
1½ cups water
2 Tbsp. soy sauce
1 Tbsp. rice vinegar
1 large clove garlic, pressed
2 tsp. fresh gingerroot, grated
1 tsp. sweetener of choice
1 Tbsp. arrowroot powder or cornstarch
½ cup scallions, chopped

1. Cut the tofu into ½" x ½" x 1" pieces.

2. Mix together the rest of the ingredients, except the arrowroot and scallions, and pour over the tofu pieces in a glass pan. Marinate, covered, overnight in the refrigerator. (If you are really in a hurry, go ahead and cook it now.)

3. Lightly spray a non-stick sauté pan with non-stick olive oil spray. Arrange the tofu pieces in a single layer, and lightly brown on both sides.

4. Mix the arrowroot into the marinade and pour over the browned tofu pieces. Gently bring to a simmer, and cook until the liquid is hot and thickened. Serve hot sprinkled with scallions.

Per serving: Calories: 134, Protein: 13 gm., Fat: 5 gm., Carbohydrates: 9 gm., Fiber 3 gm., Sodium: 509 mg.

TEXTURED VEGETABLE PROTEIN BALLS FOR PASTA AND MARINARA

Yield: 16 balls (4-6 servings)

While the TEXTURED VEGETABLE PROTEIN BALLS are baking, prepare BASIC MARINARA SAUCE, (pg. 98) or heat your favorite prepared sauce, and cook 1 lb. vermicelli or other pasta of choice according to directions. Serve hot with a MIXED GREEN SALAD (pg. 42) and crusty fat-free bread.

⅞ cup boiling water
1 cup textured vegetable protein
¼ cup unbleached white flour
1 small onion, diced, or 1 Tbsp. onion powder
1 clove garlic, minced, or ½ tsp. garlic powder
½ tsp. salt
½ tsp. oregano
¼ tsp. basil
pinch of freshly ground black pepper
1 tsp. olive oil

1. Preheat the oven to 350°F.

2. Pour the boiling water over the textured vegetable protein, and let stand for 10 minutes.

3. Fluff the soaked textured vegetable protein into a mixing bowl, and add the flour, onion, garlic, salt, oregano, basil, and black pepper. Mix all the ingredients together, and form into 16 balls.

4. Spray a non-stick baking pan with non-stick cooking spray, or oil with 1 tsp. olive oil. Arrange the balls in the pan, and bake for 30 minutes. Turn each ball every 10 minutes until lightly browned.

Per serving: Calories: 95, Protein: 9 gm., Fat: 1 gm., Carbohydrates: 12 gm., Fiber 2 gm., Sodium: 218 mg.

PITA PIZZA

YIELD: 6 INDIVIDUAL PIZZAS

This is a very popular meal or snack for children or teenagers and very easy to prepare. The ingredients can be varied according to taste. They can be prepared individually in the toaster oven or in quantity in a larger oven.

6-6" fat-free pita breads
1½ cups your favorite fat-
free pizza sauce
½ lb. firm reduced-fat
tofu, crumbled
½ green pepper, sliced
4 oz. mushrooms, sliced
3 oz. black olives, sliced
4 oz. grated fat-free soy
cheese (opt)

1. Preheat the oven to 450°F.

2. Arrange the pita breads on baking sheets. First, spread each one with the pizza sauce (about ¼ cup or to taste), then sprinkle with the tofu, mushrooms, black olives, green pepper, and grated soy cheese.

3. Bake for about 10 minutes, and serve hot.

Per pizza: Calories: 215, Protein: 15 gm., Fat: 4 gm., Carbohydrates: 37 gm., Fiber 4 gm., Sodium: 479 mg.

Burritos with Textured Vegetable Protein

Yield: Filling for 4-6 burritos (about 2½ cups)

This quick and easy filling can be used not only in burritos, but also in tostadas, enchiladas, tamales, or empanadas.

¾ cup boiling water
2 Tbsp. ketchup
1 Tbsp. chili powder
1 Tbsp. onion powder
1 tsp. salt
½ tsp. garlic powder
½ tsp. oregano
1 cup textured vegetable
    protein granules
2 tsp. olive oil
¼ cup water
1 jalapeño, minced (opt)
4-6 fat-free flour or corn
    tortillas
salsa of choice
lettuce, chopped

1. Mix together the boiling water, ketchup, chili powder, onion powder, salt, garlic powder, and oregano. Stir in the textured vegetables protein granules, and let stand for about 10 minutes.

2. Sauté the hydrated textured vegetable protein in the olive oil, with ¼ cup water and the jalapeño. Serve rolled in warmed tortillas along with your choice of salsa and lettuce.

Per burrito: Calories: 139, Protein: 10 gm., Fat: 3 gm., Carbohydrates: 19 gm., Fiber 2 gm., Sodium: 494 mg.

STUFFED ROASTED POBLANOS

YIELD: 6 SERVINGS

Poblano peppers can range from very mild to definitely picante, so beware when you bite into them. The peppers can be roasted and peeled the day before and refrigerated or even frozen until ready for use.

6 poblano peppers
2 garlic cloves
2 cups fresh cilantro leaves, lightly packed
3 Tbsp. fresh lime juice
1 tsp. salt
1 lb. reduced-fat firm tofu
1 cup tomato sauce

1. Preheat the oven to broil.

2. Always handle hot peppers with rubber gloves. I use disposable ones. Wash the peppers then roast them under the broiler, turning them until charred and blistered all over. Close the blistered peppers in a plastic or paper bag for about 15 minutes, then remove the peels, membranes, and seeds. Slit the peppers open down one side.

3. Preheat the oven to 350°F.

4. Chop the garlic in a food processor, add the cilantro leaves, and chop. Add the lime juice, salt, and tofu, and blend until creamy. Stuff each pepper with about ⅓ cup of the tofu filling. Arrange the stuffed peppers in an 11" x 7" baking dish. Pour the tomato sauce over the peppers, and bake about 35 to 40 minutes.

Per serving: Calories: 111, Protein: 9 gm., Fat: 3 gm., Carbohydrates: 11 gm., Fiber 4 gm., Sodium: 610 mg.

T-L-T Sandwich

Use BROILED TEMPEH OR TOFU (pg. 112) to build this sandwich. The tempeh or tofu will lend a bacon-like flavor.

1-6" fat-free pita bread, or
    2 slices fat-free bread
1 Tbsp. ZIPPY SALAD
    DRESSING (pg. 43)
1 tsp. mustard (or to taste)
1 serving BROILED TEMPEH OR
    TOFU (pg. 112)
4 slices tomato
2 leaves leaf lettuce

1. Open the pita bread or lay out the slices of bread. Spread with ZIPPY SALAD DRESSING and mustard, lay on the BROILED TEMPEH OR TOFU, tomato, and lettuce. Serve and enjoy.

Per sandwich: Calories: 271, Protein: 13 gm., Fat: 4 gm., Carbohydrates: 44 gm., Fiber 4 gm., Sodium: 201 mg.

TORTILLA ESPAÑOLA

YIELD: 6-8 SERVINGS

The original TORTILLA ESPAÑOLA *is made with butter, potatoes, onions, and eggs. This recipe replaces the butter with olive oil and the eggs with tofu for a reduced-fat, vegan version.*

1 Tbsp. olive oil
½ lb. onions, chopped
2 cloves garlic, minced
1 lb. potatoes
1-10.5 oz. pkg. lite silken
   tofu, or 1 lb.
   reduced-fat soft tofu
1 tsp. salt
¼ tsp. freshly ground
   black pepper

1. Preheat the oven to 350°F.

2. Sauté the onions and garlic in the olive oil until transparent.

3. Parboil the potatoes 10 minutes, peel, and grate.

4. Blend the tofu, salt, and black pepper until creamy.

5. Mix all together and pour into a lightly oiled pie pan. Bake for 45 minutes or until it starts to brown on the edges. Cut into wedges and serve.

Per serving: Calories: 102, Protein: 4 gm., Fat: 2 gm., Carbohydrates: 16 gm., Fiber 2 gm., Sodium: 349 mg.

TAMALE PIE WITH
TEXTURED VEGETABLE PROTEIN

Yield: 6-8 servings

FOR FILLING:

⅞ cup boiling water

1 cup textured vegetable
protein granules

2 tsp. olive oil

1 medium onion

1 small green pepper, or
1-4 oz. can diced green
chilies, drained

hot chile to taste

2 large tomatoes, peeled
and chopped, or
1-15 oz. can peeled,
chopped tomatoes

1 cup frozen corn

FOR CORNMEAL TOPPING:

4 cups water

1 cup cornmeal

½ tsp. garlic powder

½ tsp. salt

1. Prepare the FILLING: Pour the boiling water over the textured vegetable protein, and let set. Sauté the onion, garlic, green pepper, and chile in the olive oil. When the onion is transparent, stir in the hydrated textured vegetable protein, tomatoes, and corn. Let simmer while preparing the CORNMEAL TOPPING below.

2. Preheat the oven to 450°F.

3. Prepare the CORNMEAL TOPPING: In a 2-quart microwave-safe bowl, whip together the water, cornmeal, garlic powder, and salt. Microwave on high for 6 minutes, whip thoroughly, cover, leaving a steam escape hole, and microwave 5 more minutes. Whip thoroughly again.

4. Pour the FILLING evenly into a 2 quart casserole, and cover evenly with the CORNMEAL TOPPING. Bake for about 25 minutes or until it is browned on top.

Per serving: Calories: 164, Protein: 9 gm., Fat: 1 gm., Carbohydrates: 28 gm., Fiber 5 gm., Sodium: 162 mg.

VARIATION: Replace CORNMEAL TOPPING with CORNBREAD TOPPING: Prepare the CORNBREAD TOPPING: Mix together 1 cup cornmeal, ½ cup unbleached white flour,

1½ tsp. baking powder, and ½ tsp. salt in a mixing bowl. Make a well in the center, pour in 1 cup low-fat soymilk and 1 Tbsp. canola oil, and mix together until just moistened. Pour evenly over the *Filling* and bake for about 25 minutes or until it springs back to the touch.

Per serving: Calories: 222, Protein: 10 gm., Fat: 3 gm., Carbohydrates: 36 gm., Fiber 5 gm., Sodium: 328 mg.

TEMPEH SLOPPY JOE

YIELD: 3 CUPS (4 SERVINGS)

8 oz. tempeh
2 Tbsp. water
1 onion, chopped
1 green pepper or 2 sweet
banana peppers, chopped
2 cloves garlic, minced
2 cups BASIC MARINARA
    SAUCE, (pg. 98)
2 tsp. chili powder
½ tsp. salt

1. Steam the tempeh for 20 minutes, and cut into ¼" cubes or grate.

2. In a 1-quart microwave-safe container, cook the onion, green pepper and garlic in the water for 1 minute on high. Stir in the tempeh, BASIC MARINARA SAUCE, chili powder, and salt, and cook on high for about 2 more minutes or until heated through. Serve on toasted low-fat buns.

Per serving (sauce only): Calories: 180, Protein: 14 gm., Fat: 5 gm., Carbohydrates: 23 gm., Fiber 8 gm., Sodium: 219 mg.

Per serving (sauce and low-fat bun): Calories: 225, Protein: 16 gm., Fat: 5 gm., Carbohydrates: 32 gm., Fiber 9 gm., Sodium: 309 mg.

BROILED OR GRILLED TOFU-CARROT BURGERS

YIELD: 8 BURGERS

This is a good way to use the pulp left over from making carrot juice.

½ sweet yellow onion or
   one bunch green onions
2 cloves garlic
½ cup sunflower seeds (opt)
½ lb. firm reduced-fat tofu
2 Tbsp. sweet miso
¼ tsp. tarragon
2 cups carrots, finely grated
   or pulp from making
   carrot juice

1. In a food processor, chop the onions, garlic, and sunflower seeds. Add the tofu, miso, tarragon, and carrots, and process until blended.

2. Form into 8 burgers and broil or grill until browned on both sides. They are delicate, so handle with care. The burgers can also be fried in a small amount of oil on a non-stick surface until browned.

Per burger: Calories: 59, Protein: 4 gm., Fat: 1 gm., Carbohydrates: 7 gm., Fiber 2 gm., Sodium: 28 mg.

VEGETABLES

There is such a bountiful variety of vegetables to enjoy. The fresher they are, the better they are. Eat as many of your vegetables as you can in the raw form, while they still have all their nutrients and enzymes in tact. If you can't find them fresh, frozen is just fine. Steam your vegetables only until crisp-tender to maintain as many nutrients as possible. If you must dress your vegetables, try a drizzle of olive oil, a sprinkling of nutritional yeast, or a teaspoon of **CILANTRO-WALNUT PESTO** (pg. 48) or **BASIL-PIGNOLIA PESTO** (pg. 48), instead of butter or margarine.

Both vegetables and fruits are rich sources of antioxidants (vitamins C, E, and beta carotene), fiber, and phytochemicals which help protect the body from disease. Health experts are recommending at least 5 servings of vegetables every day. One serving is ½ cup.

The availability of new, different, and exotic types of vegetables continues to expand. Let all kinds of vegetables become a major part of your low-fat, low-calorie diet. Each one has its own unique flavor and texture for you to enjoy.

GREENS OF ALL KINDS

Allow at least ½ lb. of fresh greens per serving. One pound of fresh greens yields about one cup of cooked greens. Fresh greens are delicious, each kind having it's own distinctive, subtle flavor. Try drizzling ¼ to ½ tsp. olive oil and a sprinkling of nutritional yeast over your steamed greens. Below is a partial listing of the greens commercially available. You might find some of them in your back yard or vacant lot too! Take a chance! Try something new!

arugula or rockette
Belgian endive
beet greens
bok choy or pak choy
cabbage of all kinds
chard
collards
dandelion greens
endive or escarole
kale
lambs quarters
mizuna (mild mustard type)
mustard greens
Napa cabbage
New Zealand spinach
nettles
rapini, broccoli rabe, or raab
spinach
savoy spinach
tat-soi (an Asian type kale)
turnip greens
watercress

1. Wash and lightly steam your washed greens, only until they wilt and their color turns to a bright green (about 2 to 5 minutes). The more tender, succulent greens will take the least time. You may want to remove the stems from some of the heartier greens.

Spring and Summer Vegetables

Green Beans with Shiitake

Yield: 4-6 servings

The best flavor comes from using both fresh green beans and fresh shiitake. You can substitute frozen green beans and rehydrated dried shiitake. To rehydrate the mushrooms, pour boiling water over them, and let stand for about 20 minutes or until soft.

⅛ lb. fresh shiitake mush-
    rooms
1 tsp. sesame oil
1 lb. fresh green beans

1. Clean and slice the shiitake mushrooms about ⅛" thick, and sauté in the sesame oil over low heat until the mushrooms attain a soft, "melt in your mouth" texture. This will take anywhere from 5 to 15 minutes. (The mushrooms will exude their own liquid.)

2. Wash and trim the green beans, then steam for about 5 minutes or until crisp tender.

3. Toss all together and serve.

Per serving: Calories 43, Protein 2 gm., Fat 0 gm., Carbohydrates 7 gm., Fiber 2 gm, Sodium 5 mg.

CREAMY CURRIED POTATOES AND PEAS

YIELD: 6 CUPS (6 SERVINGS)

A colorful, mild curry to serve as a main dish or a side dish.

4 cups potatoes, cubed
   (2 lbs.)
1½ cups fresh green peas,
   or 1-9 oz. pkg. frozen
   green peas
1 tsp. oil
1 medium onion, sliced
1½ tsp. curry powder
1 Tbsp. unbleached white
   flour
1 cup low-fat soymilk
   or low-fat soy yogurt
½ tsp. salt
⅛ tsp. black pepper

1. Steam the potatoes and green peas until tender.

2. Sauté the onion in oil over low heat until transparent. Stir in the curry powder, and continue to cook over low heat for about 2 minutes, while stirring. Stir in the flour, then stir in the soymilk, salt, and black pepper, leaving no lumps.

3. Mix in the hot, steamed potatoes and green peas, and serve.

Per serving: Calories 198, Protein 5 gm., Fat 1 gm., Carbohydrates 42 gm., Fiber 5 gm, Sodium 202 mg.

KOREAN SPINACH

YIELD: 2 CUPS (ABOUT 4 SERVINGS)

Fresh spinach can be cleaned by plucking the leaves from the bunch and dropping them into a sink of clean, cold water. This eliminates having to deal with the dirt that is on the stems. Slosh the leaves around in the cold water, drain the sink, and repeat the process one or two more times until all the grit is gone. Drain the spinach in a colander. Frozen spinach can be substituted, although fresh leaves yield a better flavor and texture.

2 lbs. (2 bunches) fresh
   spinach
2 Tbsp. green onions,
   chopped
1 Tbsp. tamari
½ Tbsp. sesame seeds,
   toasted (opt)
1 large clove garlic, pressed
1 tsp. toasted sesame oil
1 tsp. sweetener of choice

1. Wash and remove the stems from the spinach. Steam over boiling water only until the leaves wilt and turn bright green.

2. Mix together the rest of the ingredients. Transfer the spinach to a serving bowl, pour the flavoring mixture over the spinach, toss, and serve.

Per serving: Calories 68, Protein 4 gm., Fat 0 gm., Carbohydrates 8 gm., Fiber 9 gm, Sodium 430 mg.

Yellow, Green, and Orange Sveltes

Yield: 4-6 servings

Flavor this dish with **Basil-Pignolia Pesto** *(pg. 48),* **Cilantro-Walnut Pesto** *(pg. 48), or other pesto of choice. This colorful side dish is featured on the cover.*

½ lb. small zucchini
½ lb. small yellow
   summer squash
½ lb. large carrot
1 small onion
1 Tbsp. Basil-Pignolia Pesto
   (pg. 48) or Cilantro-
   Walnut Pesto (pg. 48)
salt to taste

1. Wash and trim the vegetables.

2. Slice the squash and carrot lengthwise with a vegetable peeler or thin slicing blade into long, very thin strips. Cut the onion in thin slices or rounds.

3. Steam for about 3 minutes or just until tender.

4. Toss with your pesto of choice, salt to taste, and serve.

Per serving: Calories 55, Protein 1 gm., Fat 0 gm., Carbohydrates 11 gm., Fiber 3 gm, Sodium 20 mg.

Ratatouille

YIELD: 5 CUPS

This one is best at the height of summer harvest.

2 tsp. olive oil
1 medium onion, chopped
½ red bell pepper, chopped
½ green pepper, chopped
2 cloves garlic, pressed
1 lb. eggplant, cubed
2 cups plum tomatoes, chopped
1 lb. zucchini, sliced
3 Tbsp. fresh basil, minced
½ tsp. salt
⅛ tsp. freshly ground black pepper

1. Sauté all the ingredients together until the vegetables are tender. Serve hot.

Per cup: Calories 86, Protein 2 gm., Fat 1 gm., Carbohydrates 15 gm., Fiber 5 gm, Sodium 230 mg.

ARTICHOKES
WITH HONEY MUSTARD DIP

YIELD: ALLOW ONE MEDIUM ARTICHOKE PER PERSON

Artichokes are traditionally served with melted butter, butter sauces, or mayonnaise as dips. HONEY MUSTARD DIP (pg. 46) is a delicious low-fat alternative condiment for this unique vegetable. Dip each leaf, then gently pull the tender part off the leaf through your teeth, discarding the tough parts of the leaf.

1 medium artichoke per serving
HONEY MUSTARD DIP (pg. 46)

1. Wash the artichokes under cold, running water, then cut off the stem at the base. Remove any small tough bottom leaves. You can cut off about an inch of the top, and trim the prickly leaf tips, but this is not strictly necessary.

2. *Stovetop Method:* Steam over about 2 inches of boiling water, tightly covered, for about 40 minutes, adding more water if necessary. Artichokes are done when easily pierced with a fork at the base. Drain upside down. *Microwave Method:* Cover tightly and cook on high for 3 to 7 minutes per artichoke, depending on size and number. No cooking water is necessary. Let stand for about 5 minutes, then carefully release the steam.

3. Serve hot or cold with **HONEY MUSTARD DIP**.

Per serving: Calories 110, Protein 2 gm., Fat 1 gm., Carbohydrates 23 gm., Fiber 4 gm, Sodium 266 mg.

ASPARAGUS
WITH GARLIC-GINGER SAUCE

YIELD: 3-4 SERVINGS

Cook asparagus only briefly; don't let it get soggy and limp. You can peel off the tough lower skin and eat the whole stock. My favorite way to eat asparagus is fresh out of the garden, raw.

½ Tbsp. arrowroot or
    cornstarch
⅓ cup cold water
1 Tbsp. soy sauce
1 tsp. sweetener of choice
1 Tbsp. fresh gingerroot,
    peeled and grated
1 clove garlic, minced
½ tsp. toasted sesame oil
1 lb. asparagus, trimmed
    in spears
sesame seeds (opt)

1. Mix together the arrowroot, cold water, soy sauce, sweetener, gingerroot, and garlic. *Microwave Method:* In a microwave-safe bowl, microwave on high 2-3 minutes until thickened. Whip until smooth. *Stovetop Method:* Stir constantly in a saucepan over low heat a few minutes until smooth and thickened.

2. Stir in the sesame oil.

3. Steam the asparagus 1 or 2 minutes until just crisp-tender. Serve immediately with 1 to 2 tablespoons of the sauce sprinkled with sesame seeds.

Per serving: Calories 52, Protein 3 gm., Fat 0 gm., Carbohydrates 9 gm., Fiber 2 gm, Sodium 293 mg.

Grilled Vegetables

While you've got the outdoor grill going this summer, don't forget the grilled vegetables. They are a special taste treat. Grilling can be done all year round if you have a stovetop grill or an indoor electric grill.

Grilled Corn on the Cob

Yield: 6 servings

6 ears of corn, husks in tact

1. Carefully pull back the husks without removing them, remove the silk, and rinse off the ears of corn. Carefully replace the husks around the corn.

2. Grill over medium coals for about 20 minutes, turning each a quarter turn every 5 minutes.

3. Remove the husks and enjoy. Sprinkle with salt if you like.

Per serving: Calories 59, Protein 1 gm., Fat 0 gm., Carbohydrates 13 gm. Fiber 4 gm, Sodium 3 mg.

Grilled Baby Scallop Squash, Zucchini, or Summer Squash

Yield: 6 servings

6 baby scallop or pattypan squash, zucchini, or summer squash

1. Wash and trim the squash.

2. Grill over medium coals or on an electric grill about 20 minutes on each side.

Per serving: Calories 6, Protein 0 gm.. Fat 0 gm., Carbohydrates 1 gm., Fiber 0 gm, Sodium 1 mg.

GRILLED POTATOES

YIELD: ABOUT 6 SERVINGS

2-3 potatoes

1. Wash and cut the potatoes into ½" slices, and parboil about 10 minutes.

2. Grill over medium coals about 15 minutes on each side or until browned and soft.

Per serving: Calories 58, Protein 1 gm., Fat 0 gm., Carbohydrates 14 gm., Fiber 1 gm, Sodium 4 mg.

GRILLED SHIITAKE

YIELD: 6 SERVINGS

12 small or 6 medium fresh shiitake mushrooms

1. Clean and remove the stems from the mushrooms and soak in water about 10 minutes.

2. Grill, gill side up, over medium coals for about 8 to 10 minutes or until beads of liquid form on the gills.

Per serving: Calories 25, Protein 1 gm., Fat 0 gm., Carbohydrates 5 gm., Fiber 0 gm, Sodium 0 mg.

GRILLED SWEET BELL PEPPERS

YIELD: ABOUT 6 SERVINGS

2 red, yellow, or green bell peppers

1. Wash, remove seeds from peppers, and cut into 1" slices.

2. Grill over medium coals 6 to 7 minutes on each side.

Per serving: Calories 6, Protein 0 gm., Fat 0 gm., Carbohydrates 1 gm., Fiber 0 gm, Sodium 1 mg.

VEGETABLE GUMBO

YIELD: 6 CUPS

This light version of Gumbo still has all the flavor.

1 tsp. olive oil
1 large onion, chopped
1 green pepper, chopped
2 ribs celery, chopped
1 lb. zucchini, sliced
6 oz. okra, sliced
2 cloves garlic, minced or
   pressed
1 cup parsley, chopped
1 bay leaf
½ tsp. thyme
½ tsp. oregano
½ tsp. salt
⅛ tsp. cayenne
1 Tbsp. olive oil
2 Tbsp. unbleached white
   flour
1-16 oz. can diced
   tomatoes

1. Sauté the onion, green pepper, celery, zucchini, okra, and garlic in the 1 tsp. olive oil until the onion starts to turn translucent. Add a little water if it starts to stick. Add the parsley, bay leaf, thyme, oregano, salt, and cayenne, cover, and steam until tender.

2. In a small saucepan, mix together the 1 Tbsp. olive oil and the unbleached white flour. Let them bubble together over low heat until golden. Stir in the diced tomatoes, then pour over the hot vegetables. Toss, remove the bay leaf, and serve with rice.

Per cup: Calories 92, Protein 2 gm., Fat 2 gm., Carbohydrates 13 gm., Fiber 4 gm, Sodium 204 mg.

Fall and Winter Vegetables

Butternut Squash Stuffed with Spiced Pears

Yield: 2-4 servings

A mixture or savory and sweet flavors that can be served as a main dish or a side dish.

1 medium butternut squash
   or 2 small ones
   (about 2 lbs.)
1 tsp. canola oil
½ cup onion, finely
   chopped
2 pears, cored and diced
1 Tbsp. apple juice
2 Tbsp. sweetener of choice
1 tsp. fresh gingerroot,
   minced, or ⅛ tsp. dried
   ginger
⅛ tsp. cinnamon
pinch of allspice or cloves
2 Tbsp. roasted, slivered
   almonds (opt)

1. Preheat the oven to 350°F.

2. Wash the squash, cut it in half, and scoop out the seeds. Bake, cut side down, in a shallow baking pan until almost tender (about 40 minutes).

3. While the squash is baking, sauté the onion in the canola oil until transparent, then mix in the pears, apple juice, sweetener, gingerroot, cinnamon, and allspice. Cook gently for 3 to 4 minutes. Spoon the filling into the scooped out hole in the almost tender squash, and sprinkle with slivered almonds. Return to the oven for about 10 more minutes or until tender.

Per serving: Calories 249, Protein 3 gm., Fat 2 gm., Carbohydrates 52 gm., Fiber 12 gm, Sodium 5 mg.

STEAMED "STIR-FRIED" VEGETABLES

YIELD: 2-4 SERVINGS

Here are tender, tasty "stir-fried" vegetables without the fat. Have all the vegetables cut to size before you start cooking. Cook the vegetables just to crisp-tender. You can use any combination of vegetables you like or have on hand. Vary the flavoring according to taste.

½ lb. broccoli
½ large onion
½ red bell pepper
½ yellow bell pepper
½ lb. yellow summer
   squash
½ cup water
½ Tbsp. soy sauce
2 cloves garlic, minced
1 tsp. fresh gingerroot,
   grated

1. Wash and cut all the vegetables to the same size and thickness for equal cooking time.

2. Pour the water, soy sauce, garlic, and gingerroot into a wok or other deep pan with a tight fitting lid. Bring to a boil and add the broccoli. Cover tightly and steam for 2 to 3 minutes.

3. Open the lid, stir in all the other ingredients, cover, and steam 2 more minutes, until the vegetables are crisp-tender. Serve immediately.

Per serving: Calories 55, Protein 2 gm., Fat 0 gm., Carbohydrates 10 gm., Fiber 4 gm, Sodium 191 mg.

BASQUE WINTER VEGETABLE STEW

YIELD: 10 CUPS

This savory stew can be served as a main dish with some greens or a salad on the side.

1 Tbsp. olive oil
2 large cloves garlic, crushed
1 medium onion, chopped
2 leeks, sliced (white part only)
1 large carrot, sliced (about 1 cup)
2 potatoes, cubed (about 2 cups)
1 rutabaga, cubed (about 2 cups)
1 cup water
1 bay leaf
½ cabbage, thinly sliced (about 8 cups)
1-16 oz. can white beans
1 tsp. salt
¼ tsp. thyme
¼ cup fresh parsley, chopped
¼ tsp. freshly ground black pepper

1. In a 4-quart pot, briefly sauté the garlic, onion, leeks, carrot, potatoes, and rutabaga in the olive oil. Add the water and bay leaf, cover, and simmer gently for about 15 minutes.

2. Add the cabbage, white beans, salt, and thyme, cover, and simmer gently for about 15 minutes or until the vegetables are tender.

3. Add the parsley and black pepper, and simmer for a few more minutes. Serve hot.

Per cup: Calories 161, Protein 5 gm., Fat 1 gm., Carbohydrates 30 gm., Fiber 6 gm, Sodium 266 mg.

ROASTED ROOT VEGETABLES

Roasting caramelizes and concentrates the natural sugars in root vegetables which results in a golden crisp skin and a moist but "meaty" texture inside. Try crumbling thyme, rosemary, or chives over the vegetables for a variation. A convection roasting setting on the oven will speed up the cooking time. Allow about ½ lb. of vegetables per serving.

CHOOSE ANY COMBINATION:
white potatoes
rutabagas
carrots
turnips
parsnips
sweet potatoes
yams
onions
garlic
shallots
1 tsp. oil per every ½ lb.
    vegetables (opt)
salt to taste

1. Preheat the oven to 400°F.

2. Wash the vegetables and cut into 1½" chunks. Cut the carrots and rutabagas a little smaller; they take the longest to roast.

2. Rub the vegetables with the oil and arrange them in a roasting pan so that they are not crowded together. Sprinkle with salt. If you are going to roast garlic, don't add it to the pan until the last 20 minutes of roasting.

3. Roast the vegetables uncovered, for about 40 to 50 minutes, turning about every 15 minutes. If they start to look as if they will burn on the edges before they are done inside, lower the heat to 350°F, or cover tightly with aluminum foil. Carrots, rutabagas, and white potatoes will take the longest to roast.

Per serving: Calories 195, Protein 3 gm., Fat 0 gm., Carbohydrates 46 gm., Fiber 5 gm, Sodium 12 mg.

CURRIED CARROT, TURNIP, AND ONION

Serve as a side dish or over brown rice topped with soy yogurt for a main dish. Other vegetables can be substituted; use what you have on hand.

½ lb. carrots, grated
½ lb. turnips, grated
1 tsp. canola oil
1 Tbsp. water
½ onion, grated (about ½ cup)
2 tsp. fresh curry powder
¼ cup fresh cilantro, chopped
½ tsp. salt

1. Steam the carrots and turnips for about 5 minutes. Reserve the steaming water.

2. Sauté the onion in the canola oil and water over low heat until soft, then stir in the curry powder. Stir and simmer about 2 minutes, then stir in the steamed vegetables, cilantro, about ½ cup of the steaming water, and salt.

Per cup: Calories 27, Protein 0 gm., Fat 1 gm., Carbohydrates 4 gm., Fiber 1 gm, Sodium 282 mg.

MASHED RUTABAGA

YIELD: ABOUT 2 CUPS

Rutabagas have a sweet, fresh taste and offer an interesting change from potatoes.

1½ lbs. rutabagas
1 Tbsp. fresh parsley
¼ tsp. salt

1. Peel the rutabagas and grate in a food processor.

2. Steam for 5 to 8 minutes until soft, then purée in a food processor along with the parsley and salt. Serve hot, as you would mashed potatoes.

Per serving: Calories 58, Protein 2 gm., Fat 0 gm., Carbohydrates 12 gm., Fiber 3 gm, Sodium 164 mg.

WINTER VEGETABLE HASH

YIELD: 3 CUPS

This is especially quick and easy if you do your grating in the food processor.

1 tsp. olive oil
½ onion, finely chopped
1 small red or green bell
   pepper, finely chopped
4 cups winter vegetables
   (turnip, rutabaga, carrot,
   cabbage, etc.), grated
salt and freshly ground black
   pepper to taste

1. Briefly sauté the onion and bell pepper in the olive oil, and stir in the grated vegetables.

2. Cover tightly and let steam for about 10 minutes or until crisp-tender. Season with salt and black pepper to taste.

Per serving: Calories 92, Protein 1 gm., Fat 1 gm., Carbohydrates 18 gm., Fiber 4 gm, Sodium 52 mg.

NORTH AFRICAN SQUASH

A different seasoning twist for winter squash.

2 lbs. winter squash, peeled, seeded, and cut into 1" cubes
¾ cup water
4 cloves garlic, pressed
1 tsp. fresh gingerroot, grated
1 tsp. salt
¼ tsp. freshly ground black pepper
6 Tbsp. fresh lemon juice
2 Tbsp. fresh cilantro, chopped
⅛ tsp. cayenne

1. In a covered pan, simmer the squash, water, garlic, gingerroot, salt, and black pepper gently together, until tender. Stir occasionally to keep from sticking.

2. When the squash is tender, sprinkle with lemon juice, cilantro, and cayenne, toss, and serve.

Per serving: Calories 78, Protein 1 gm., Fat 0 gm., Carbohydrates 16 gm., Fiber 5 gm, Sodium 429 mg.

Rutabaga Latke

This is a lighter version of the usually heavily fried potato latke. You can replace the rutabagas with grated, parboiled potatoes.

¾ lb. rutabagas, grated
½ onion, grated
2 cloves garlic, minced
1-10.5 oz. pkg. lite silken
    tofu
salt to taste
freshly ground black pepper
    to taste
2 tsp. canola or olive oil

1. Preheat the oven to 450°F.

2. Mix together the rutabagas, onion, and garlic.

3. In a blender or food processor, blend the tofu, salt, and black pepper until creamy.

4. Spread a non-stick cookie sheet with the canola oil. Shape the mixture into 12 latkes on the sheet. Bake for about 10 minutes, carefully turn the latkes, and bake 5 more minutes. Serve hot.

Per latke: Calories: 23, Protein: 2 gm., Fat: 0 gm., Carbohydrates: 3 gm., Fiber: 1 gm, Sodium: 29 mg.

LIGHTER SWEET THINGS

In a low-fat life-style, sweet things are not meant to accompany every meal, but are special, occasional treats. Sweet, creamy, fudgy, and gooey things do not have to disappear from you life to maintain a healthy diet. All of these recipes have had the sweetener and oil reduced from the levels in conventional recipes but are still sweet and flavorful.

I have left the type of sweetener to be used up to you. There are so many different opinions and theories about sweeteners as well as individual sensitivity. You decide what and how much you want to use. These recipes give you some guidelines for reduced sweetener consumption.

LIGHTER PIES, CAKES, TARTS, AND COOKIES

LEMON TOFU CHEESECAKE

YIELD: ONE 9" SPRING FORM PAN (8-12 SERVINGS)

Featured on the cover topped with FRESH MANGO SAUCE (pg. 151), this luscious treat has a creamy texture and a delicate flavor. It is easy to prepare. Try using fresh lime juice and zest for a variation in flavor.

FOR THE CRUST:
1¼ cups graham cracker crumbs (about 10 crackers)
2 Tbsp. melted margarine
¼ cup granulated sweetener

FOR THE FILLING:
2-10.5 oz. pkgs. lite silken tofu
6 Tbsp. fresh lemon juice
½ cup sweetener of choice
2 tsp. organic lemon zest
1 tsp. vanilla

1. Preheat the oven to 350°F.

2. Prepare the CRUST: In a food processor, blend together the graham crackers, margarine, and sweetener. Pat into a 9" spring form pan

3. Prepare the FILLING: In a food processor, blend together the tofu, lemon juice, sweetener, lemon zest, and vanilla. Pour the filling into the prepared crust, and bake for about 45 minutes or until small cracks start to form around the edges of the cheesecake.

4. Let cool, cut, and serve topped with FRESH MANGO SAUCE (pg. 151), fresh fruit, fruit filling, or CREAMY TOFU TOPPING (pg. 151).

Per serving: Calories: 119, Protein: 5 gm., Fat: 3 gm., Carbohydrates: 18 gm., Fiber: 0 gm., Sodium: 99 mg..

APPLE-CRANBERRY-ORANGE TART

YIELD: ONE 9" TART (6-8 SERVINGS)

A flavorful, sweet, and tangy tart.

FOR THE **CRUST:**
1 cup whole wheat pastry
   flour
2 Tbsp. oil
¼ cup cold water

FOR THE **FILLING:**
1 lb. tart green apples,
   peeled, cored, and thinly
   sliced (about 4 cups)
1 cup cranberries, washed
   and sorted
1½ Tbsp. organic orange
   zest
¼ cup orange juice (juice
   from one small orange)
½ cup sweetener of choice
1 tsp. cinnamon
2 Tbsp. unbleached white
   flour

1. Prepare the **CRUST:** Process the flour and oil in a food processor until the consistency of cornmeal. While the processor is running, pour in the cold water. Process only long enough for the dough to start to form a ball. Gather the dough into a ball, and roll out to fit a 9" tart pan, handling as little as possible.

2. Preheat the oven to 350°F.

3. Prepare the **FILLING:** Arrange the apple slices and cranberries in the tart pan lined with the unbaked crust. Mix the rest of the ingredients together, and pour over all. Bake for 45 minutes to one hour or until the apple slices are tender. Serve hot or cold.

Per serving: Calories: 147, Protein: 3 gm., Fat: 3 gm., Carbohydrates: 24 gm., Fiber: 5 gm., Sodium: 2 mg.

FRESH BLUEBERRY TOFU CREAM PIE

YIELD: ONE 9" PIE (6-8 SERVINGS)

Substitute frozen blueberries if you can't find fresh ones.

FOR THE CRUST:
1 cup whole wheat pastry
  flour
2 Tbsp. oil
¼ cup cold water

FOR THE FILLING:
1-10.5 oz. pkg. lite silken
  tofu
¼ cup unbleached white
  flour
½ cup fructose or sweetener
  of choice
1 tsp. vanilla
¼ tsp. salt
3 cups fresh blueberries

1. Preheat the oven to 350°F.

2. Prepare the CRUST: Process the flour and oil in a food processor until it is the consistency of cornmeal. While the processor is running, pour in the cold water. Process only long enough for the dough to start to form a ball. Gather the dough into a ball, and roll out to fit a 9" pan. Press into place if you need to.

3. Prepare the FILLING: Blend the tofu, flour, sweetener, vanilla, and salt in a food processor or blender. Fold in the blueberries and pour into the unbaked 9" pastry shell. Bake for 45 minutes, cool, and serve.

Per serving: Calories: 233, Protein: 6 gm., Fat: 4 gm., Carbohydrates: 42 gm., Fiber: 4 gm., Sodium: 123 mg.

ORANGE-CARROT-SPICE CAKE

YIELD: ONE BUNDT CAKE (24 SLICES)

A moist, sweet, spicy blend of flavors. Drizzle optional LEMON GLAZE *(pg. 150) over the top of the cooled cake. You can use fresh grated carrots or the pulp left from making carrot juice to make this cake.*

2 cups unbleached white flour
2 cups whole wheat flour
1½ tsp. baking powder
1½ tsp. baking soda
2 tsp. cinnamon
½ tsp. allspice
¼ tsp. nutmeg
½ tsp. salt
¼ cup oil
1½ cups sweetener of choice
1¾ cups orange juice
2 Tbsp. organic orange zest
1 Tbsp. fresh gingerroot, finely chopped
¾ lb. carrots, grated
½ cup raisins (opt)
½ cup walnuts, chopped (opt)

1. Preheat the oven to 350°F.

2. Mix all the dry ingredients together.

3. In a mixer, mix together the oil, sweetener, orange juice, orange zest, and gingerroot until smooth and creamy.

4. Add the dry ingredients to the wet mixture, and beat until smooth. Beat in the carrots, raisins, and walnuts.

5. Pour into a non-stick bundt pan sprayed with non-stick spray, and bake for 45 to 50 minutes. Let cool about 15 minutes before removing from the pan. When cool, drizzle with LEMON GLAZE (pg. 150).

Per slice: Calories: 176, Protein: 2 gm., Fat: 2 gm., Carbohydrates: 35 gm., Fiber: 2 gm., Sodium: 6 mg..

APPLE PIZZA

YIELD: ONE 12" PIE (8 SLICES)

Apples can be replaced by any hard fruit or berry in season. Try drizzling LEMON GLAZE (pg. 150) over the cooled pie.

FOR THE CRUST:
¼ cup sweetener of choice
⅓ cup warm water
½ Tbsp. active dry yeast
1 Tbsp. oil (opt)
1½ cups unbleached white
    flour or whole wheat
    pastry flour
¼ tsp. salt

FOR THE FILLING:
3-4 lbs. apples, thinly sliced
    (6 cups)
2 Tbsp. fresh lemon juice
¼ cup sweetener of choice
1 Tbsp. unbleached white
    flour
1 tsp. cinnamon

1. Prepare the **CRUST:** In a mixer bowl or food processor bowl, dissolve the sweetener in warm water, then sprinkle the yeast on top. Let stand until foaming. Mix in the oil, flour, and salt, and knead until smooth. Place the kneaded dough in an oiled bowl, and let rise until double. While the dough is rising, prepare the **FILLING** below. When the dough is doubled, punch down and roll out to fit a 12" pizza pan.

2. Preheat the oven to 400°F.

3. Prepare the **FILLING:** Wash peel, core, and slice the apples into thin slices. Mix the slices together with the rest of the ingredients. Spread the filling over the crust, and bake about 15 minutes until the crust is browned and the apples are soft. Serve hot or cold.

Per slice: Calories: 242, Protein: 4 gm., Fat: 0 gm., Carbohydrates: 55 gm., Fiber: 4 gm., Sodium: 68 mg.

FUDGY COCOA MINT COOKIES

YIELD: 48 COOKIES

Zucchini helps make these fudgy, chewy cookies moist. They are moister and chewier the second day, if they last that long. Vanilla, coffee, or coconut extract can be substituted for the peppermint.

3 cups unbleached or whole wheat flour or half and half of each
¾ cup cocoa
2 tsp. baking soda
¼ tsp. salt
2 Tbsp. oil
1½ cups granulated sweetener
1 tsp. peppermint extract
2½ cups zucchini, finely grated (⅜ lb.)
1 cup broken walnuts (opt)

1. Preheat the oven to 350°F.

2. Mix the flour, cocoa, baking soda, and salt together in a bowl.

3. Beat the oil, sweetener, zucchini, and peppermint extract together with a mixer. Add the dry ingredients and beat until smooth. Fold in the walnuts.

4. Drop by tablespoonful onto cookie sheets, and bake for about 12 minutes.

Per cookie: Calories: 57, Protein: 1 gm., Fat: 1 gm., Carbohydrates: 12 gm., Fiber: 1 gm., Sodium: 65 mg.

LIGHTER SWEET TOPPINGS

LEMON GLAZE

YIELD: 1 CUP

2 cups confectioners sugar
¼ cup fresh lemon juice

1. Stir the ingredients together, and drizzle over cake or pastry.

Per 2 Tbsp.: Calories: 112, Protein: 0 gm., Fat: 0 gm., Carbohydrates: 30 gm., Fiber: 0 gm., Sodium: 0 mg.

COCOA SYRUP

YIELD: 1¼ CUPS

Use this syrup to flavor drinks or drizzle over desserts.

1 cup sugar
½ cup cocoa
½ cup water
1 tsp. vanilla

1. Whip together the sugar, cocoa, and water in a 1-quart glass measuring cup. Microwave 2 minutes. Let the bubbles settle down, and microwave 2 more minutes.

2. Stir in the vanilla. Serve hot or let cool. Refrigerate in a covered jar. Keeps in the refrigerator for several weeks.

Per 2 Tbsp.: Calories: 90, Protein 1 gm., Fat 0 gm., Carbohydrates 20 gm., Fiber 2 gm., Sodium: 2 mg.

FRESH MANGO SAUCE

YIELD: 1 CUP

Pour this tangy, tropical sauce over LEMON TOFU CHEESECAKE *(pg. 144), featured on the cover.*

1 ripe mango, peeled,
  pitted, and chopped
  (about 1 cup)
1 Tbsp. fresh lime juice
1 Tbsp. sweetener of choice

1. Blend all the ingredients together in a blender until creamy smooth. Serve at room temperature for full flavor.

Per 2 Tbsp.: Calories: 23, Protein: 0 gm., Fat: 0 gm., Carbohydrates: 5 gm., Fiber: 1 gm., Sodium: 0 mg.

CREAMY TOFU TOPPING

YIELD: 1½ CUPS

This is a creamy, low-fat replacement for whipped cream.

1-10.5 oz. pkg. lite silken
  tofu
¼ cup fructose or sweetener
  of choice
1 tsp. vanilla extract

1. Blend all the ingredients together in a food processor or blender until smooth and creamy. Serve chilled or at room temperature.

Per 2 Tbsp.: Calories: 25, Protein: 2 gm., Fat: 0 gm., Carbohydrates: 4 gm., Fiber: 0 gm., Sodium: 23 mg.

FRUIT TREATS

STRAWBERRY SORBET

YIELD: 10 CUPS

Here is a sweet, light, icy treat with enticing red color.

2 Tbsp. kanten
1½ cups water
1 cup sweetener of choice
    (this may vary depend
    ing on the sweetness of
    the berries)
8 cups fresh strawberries

1. Soak the kanten and water together for 10 to 15 minutes in a large glass measuring cup.

2. Stir in the sweetener until dissolved. Microwave on high 3 to 4 minutes until boiling, and let cool. Blend in a food processor with the strawberries.

3. Churn-freeze the mixture in an ice cream machine according to machine's directions. (It took 20 minutes in my machine.) The frozen mixture can be molded. The mold should be either packed in salted ice or put in the freezer for about 3 hours before use. Remove from the mold about 5 minutes before serving.

Per cup: Calories: 109, Protein: 1 gm., Fat: 0 gm., Carbohydrates: 26 gm., Fiber: 2 gm., Sodium: 2 mg.

GINGER-PEACH DUMPLINGS

YIELD: 8-10 SERVINGS

Tangy fresh ginger adds a new zest to sweet, ripe peaches. Some people would call this a "grunt," but a this method was described to me by a real southern lady as dumplings.

FOR THE *FILLING*:

6 cups sliced peaches
2 Tbsp. fresh lemon juice
¾ cup brown sugar or
   sweetener of choice
2 tsp. fresh gingerroot,
   finely chopped
½ cup water
1 Tbsp. arrowroot or corn
   starch

FOR THE *DUMPLINGS*:

1½ cups unbleached white
   flour
2 Tbsp. granulated
   sweetener of choice
2 tsp. baking powder
½ tsp. baking soda
2 Tbsp. oil
½ cup low-fat soymilk

1. Preheat the oven to 400°F.

2. Prepare the *FILLING*: In a mixing bowl, mix together the peaches, lemon juice, sweetener, and gingerroot. In a smaller bowl, mix together the water and arrowroot. Pour the starch mixture over the peach mixture, and gently mix together.

3. Prepare the *DUMPLINGS:* Mix together the flour, granulated sweetener, baking powder, and baking soda. Mix the oil and soymilk together, then mix gently into the dry ingredients just until a soft dough forms. Roll the dumpling dough out on a lightly floured board to ⅛" thick. Cut into eight 1½" strips to fit the baking pan.

4. Pour half of the peach mixture into a 2-quart baking pan. Lay half the dumpling strips over the first layer of peaches, pour the rest of the peach mixture over them, then lay the rest of the strips on top. Bake for about 20 minutes or until browned on top and the fruit is tender. Serve hot or cold. Top with CREAMY TOFU TOPPING (pg. 151) if you like.

Per serving: Calories: 207, Protein: 3 gm., Fat: 3 gm., Carbohydrates: 42 gm., Fiber: 2 gm., Sodium: 150 mg.

STRAWBERRY BISQUE

YIELD: 2 CUPS (4 SERVINGS)

Sweet and creamy and very quick and easy, this bisque can be served as an appetizer or a dessert. Add a sprig of mint to serve.

**2 cups fresh or frozen
strawberries
2 Tbsp. sweetener of choice
½-10.5 oz. pkg. lite silken
tofu**

1. Blend all the ingredients together in a blender until smooth and creamy. Chill and serve.

Per serving: Calories: 60, Protein: 3 gm., Fat: 1 gm., Carbohydrates: 11 gm., Fiber: 2 gm., Sodium: 36 mg..

FRESH AND DRIED FRUIT

YIELD: WHATEVER YOU LIKE

Nature's own sweet treat comes in the form of fruit. Fresh fruit in season is the best. Most fruit is virtually fat-free and is a good source of vitamin C, A, and potassium. Try some of the exotic new fruits that are available in your local supermarkets. Squirt fresh lemon juice over cut fruit to keep it from turning brown. GINGER-CINNAMON DIP (pg. 14) makes a tasty topping for a cup of fruit.

Dried fruits are concentrated, energy-lifting, low-fat treats which are also a source of potassium, iron, and fiber. If you are on the move, they travel well.

SMOOTHIES

Smoothies can be served for breakfast, brunch, snacks, or dessert. Use any combination of fresh or frozen fruit and fruit juices that appeal to you. This is a good use for any bananas that get ripe before anyone is ready to eat them. Peel them, seal in a freezer bag, and freeze. They add a creamy thickness to smoothies.

MANGO-BANANA-STRAWBERRY SMOOTHIE

YIELD: ABOUT 4 CUPS

2 small frozen bananas
1 large fresh mango, cut off
  the seed (about 1½ cups)
1 cup strawberries
1 cup apple or orange juice

1. Break the bananas in pieces. Blend all the ingredients together in a blender until smooth and creamy.

Per cup: Calories: 125, Protein: 1 gm., Fat: 0 gm., Carbohydrates: 29 gm., Fiber: 3 gm., Sodium: 6 mg..

BLUEBERRY-BANANA-PEACH SMOOTHIE

YIELD: 2 CUPS

1 frozen banana
1 cup frozen blueberries
1 cup apple juice or papaya
  concentrate
½ cup frozen peaches

1. Break the banana in pieces. Blend all the ingredients together in a blender until smooth and creamy.

Per cup: Calories: 166, Protein: 1 gm., Fat: 1 gm., Carbohydrates: 38 gm., Fiber: 4 gm., Sodium: 10 mg..

INDEX

Ask your store to carry these books, or you may order directly from:

The Book Publishing Company   Or call: 1-800-695-2241
P.O. Box 99 Summertown, TN 38483   Please add $2.50 per book for shipping